Planning for Pregnancy, Birth, and Beyond

The American College of
Obstetricians and Gynecologists

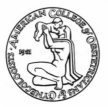

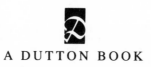

A DUTTON BOOK

Designed as an aid to patients, *Planning for Pregnancy, Birth, and Beyond* sets forth current information and opinions on subjects related to women's health and reproduction. The information does not dictate an exclusive course of treatment or procedure to be followed and should not be construed as excluding other medical opinions or acceptable methods of practice. Variations taking into account the needs of the individual patient, resources, and limitations unique to the institution or type of practice may be appropriate.

DUTTON
Published by the Penguin Group
Penguin Books USA Inc., 375 Hudson Street, New York, New York 10014, U.S.A.
Penguin Books Ltd, 27 Wrights Lane, London W8 5TZ, England
Penguin Books Australia Ltd, Ringwood, Victoria, Australia
Penguin Books Canada Ltd, 10 Alcorn Avenue, Toronto, Ontario, Canada M4V 3B2
Penguin Books (N.Z.) Ltd, 182-190 Wairau Road, Auckland 10, New Zealand

Penguin Books Ltd, Registered Offices: Harmondsworth, Middlesex, England

Published by Dutton, an imprint of New American Library,
a division of Penguin Books USA Inc.
Distributed in Canada by McClelland & Stewart Inc.

First Dutton Printing, May, 1992
10 9 8 7 6 5 4 3 2 1

Previously published as *ACOG Guide to Planning for Pregnancy, Birth, and Beyond*.

REGISTERED TRADEMARK—MARCA REGISTRADA

LIBRARY OF CONGRESS CATALOGING-IN-PUBLICATION DATA:
Planning for pregnancy, birth, and beyond / American College of
    Obstetricians and Gynecologists.
        p.   cm.
    Rev. ed. of: ACOG guide to planning for pregnancy, birth, and
beyond. c1990.
    ISBN 0-525-93473-1
    1. Pregnancy.   2. Childbirth.   3. Infants—Care. I. American
College of Obstetricians and Gynecologists.   II. ACOG guide to
planning for pregnancy, birth, and beyond.
RG556.P53   1992
618.2'4—dc20   91-42702
                                            CIP

Printed in the United States of America
Set in Times Roman
Designed by Esther Millen Smail

Acknowledgments

Planning for Pregnancy, Birth, and Beyond was developed under the direction of the Division of Education and the American College of Obstetricians and Gynecologists by a panel of consultants who represent various levels of ACOG and NAACOG (the Nurses' Association of ACOG) leadership, geographic areas, and types of practice.

Editors
Harrison C. Visscher, MD, FACOG
Rebecca D. Rinehart

Associate Editors
Mary F. Harris
Kathleen E. Achor

Consultants
Ronald A. Chaz, MD, FACOG
Fredric Frigoletto, MD, FACOG
William K. Graves, MD, FACOG

Sherry L. M. Jimenez, RN, ACCE
George A. Little, MD, FAAP, FACOG
Rebecca Shaw, MD, FACOG

In addition to the consultants, other contributors and reviewers are gratefully acknowledged:

Constance J. Bohon, MD, FACOG
Sheila E. Cohen, MD, ASA
Sharon L. Dooley, MD, FACOG
Sherman Elias, MD, FACOG
Jeffrey Greenspan, MD, FACOG

Carla Harris, RNC, MSN
Carol L. C. Little, MD, FAAP
Elizabeth M. Ramsey, MD, FACOG
Sallye Shaw, RN, MN
Carl W. Tyler, Jr., MD, FACOG

Illustration
Marilyn Kaufman
Lidia Kibiuk
Mary B. Marine
Lois Sloan

Terese Winslow
John Yanson
Patricia Tobin

Photography
Earl Dotter, © Earl Dotter
Marjorie M. Pyle, RNC, ACCE, © Lifecircle; taken at Los Alamitos Medical Center, Los Alamitos, CA

Contents

Preface

Congratulations! By opening this book, you have just taken an important step toward a healthy pregnancy. The American College of Obstetricians and Gynecologists (ACOG), the national medical organization devoted to women's health care, has assembled in one book what a woman should know about her pregnancy—before, during, and afterward—to enable her to take an active role in her health care. Designed for women who are pregnant or planning to become pregnant, *Planning for Pregnancy, Birth, and Beyond* is ACOG's complete guide to preconception, prenatal, and postpartum care. It presents current, scientifically accurate information about what to expect from your health care team and what you can do to improve your chances of having a healthy baby.

Planning for Pregnancy, Birth, and Beyond begins with preconception care—that important time before a pregnancy begins when a woman's health and life style can have a major impact on her fetus—and continues through the changes that occur over the 9 months of pregnancy. It concludes with a step-by-step description of labor and delivery with detailed information on what to expect after you and your baby go home. The latest advances in areas such as prenatal testing and fetal assessment are presented, along with practical information on your general health and well-being in areas such as nutrition, exercise, work, and relationships.

Planning for Pregnancy, Birth, and Beyond is a reference to all aspects of pregnancy, including those that relate to special needs or problems. The information is organized to help you turn to or skip a particular area, with cross-references to related subjects. The complete subject index at the back can help you locate topics of interest. Other features include an extensive glossary, which defines terms marked by **boldface italic** letters at first mention, and a personal pregnancy diary that can be used to chart the progress of your pregnancy and to note key events. Questions at the end of each chapter reinforce important concepts and form the basis for a dialogue between you and your doctor.

The information in this book represents the opinions of leading experts in the specialty and related fields and is drawn from educational materials developed by ACOG for practicing obstetrician–gynecologists. The views expressed here are not absolute, however, and should be considered flexible guidelines based on the advice of your doctor and the limitations of resources in your community.

Pregnancy is not an illness, but sometimes illness occurs with or is caused by pregnancy. Although advances in prenatal care have markedly improved the outcome for mothers and babies, there are no guarantees in medicine. Pregnancy is a normal, natural process for most women, however, that always has a profound impact on those it touches. Working together, you and your doctor can direct your efforts toward the goal of pregnancy—the delivery of a healthy baby.

Section I

Preconception Care

Section I

Preconception Care

Becoming a parent is a major commitment filled with challenges, rewards, and choices. By making some plans and adjustments now, you will promote a healthy pregnancy later. Some aspects of pregnancy are part of the natural process over which you have no control. However, you can control one of the most important factors in determining your health and that of your baby—your life style. Planning for pregnancy in advance can help prepare you for the experience ahead and help promote a healthy life style for your future.

Chapter 1

Planning Your Pregnancy

Pregnancy is a major event. When it is planned in advance, a woman can make decisions that will benefit both her health and that of her baby. Good general health before pregnancy can help you cope with the stress of pregnancy, labor, and delivery. It can also help ensure that neither you nor your baby is exposed to things that could be harmful.

Many women do not know they are pregnant until 5, 6, or even 8 weeks. About 2 weeks after a woman's menstrual cycle, an egg can be fertilized by a man's sperm; it then moves to a woman's uterus and becomes attached there to grow. These early weeks are some of the most significant ones for the baby, because it is during this time that the baby's body and internal organs are formed. Certain substances—for example, alcohol, cigarettes, and drugs—may interfere with that growth, whereas a healthy life style may help promote it. Preconception, or prepregnancy, care can guide you in planning for a healthy pregnancy.

A Preconception Visit

You may wish to arrange a special visit with your doctor to discuss your plans for pregnancy. As part of your preconception visit, you will be asked questions about your medical history, any past pregnancies, and your life style. The answers to

3

Preconception Care Inventory

Patient name _____ Age_____ Husband _____
Patient address _____ Telephone _____
Referring physician _____
Referring physician address _____ Telephone _____
Religion _____ Ethnic background _____ Blood type _____
Receives regular health care by _____
Reason for seeking preconception counseling _____
_____

Family history

_____ Diabetes (relationship to patient) _____
_____ Hypertension (relationship to patient) _____
_____ Epilepsy (relationship to patient) _____
_____ Multiple pregnancies (relationship to patient) _____
_____ Other (specify) _____

Genetic history

Has the patient been screened for special disease relating to ethnic background?
_____ yes _____ no   If yes, explain _____
Is there any family history of: (Include previous children by either parent)
_____ Muscular dystrophy (relationship to patient) _____
_____ Hemophilia (relationship to patient) _____
_____ Cystic fibrosis (relationship to patient) _____
_____ Mental retardation (relationship to patient) _____
_____ Birth defects (relationship to patient) _____
_____ Short stature (relationship to patient) _____
Is there anything that the patient is especially concerned about? _____
_____
_____
_____

Medical history

_____ Diabetes: Onset? _____
_____ Hypertension: Onset? _____ Range? _____
_____ Epilepsy: Onset? _____
_____ Anemia: For how long? _____
_____ Rubella: When? _____
_____ Menses: Onset? _____ Regular _____
_____ Surgery: If so, what type? _____
_____ Contraception: Methods used? _____
_____ Accidents: What type? _____
_____ Allergies: What type? _____
_____ Immunizations: _____

Current medication

General: (including over-the-counter drugs) _____
_____

Preconception Care Inventory *(continued)*

Specific:
_____ Oral contraceptives: Type _____ Duration _____
_____ Sedatives or Tranquilizers: _____
_____ Drugs: _____
_____ Alcohol: _____ Beer _____ Wine _____ Liquor _____
_____ Smoking: _____ Packs per day _____
_____ Snuff: _____
_____ Appetite suppressants: _____
_____ Diuretics: _____
_____ Antibiotics: _____
_____ Caffeine: _____

Nutrition

Present status:
Height _____ Weight _____
Does the patient make an effort to control weight?   _____ yes _____ no
Does the patient take vitamins?   _____ yes _____ no
If yes, which ones? _____
Is the patient a vegetarian?   _____ yes _____ no
If yes, what type? _____

Environmental factors

Occupation _____
Hobbies _____
Source of water supply _____
Pets _____ Exercise _____

Obstetric history

Gravida _____ Para _____
Deliveries _____ Management _____
Surgery _____
Pregnancy complications _____

Counseling

Specialized _____

Comments

_____
_____

This information may be discussed during a preconception visit.

these questions should be honest and open. They will let your doctor know whether you may need special care during pregnancy, and they will be treated as confidential information.

Some women have medical conditions that require special attention or care during pregnancy. The condition may be an illness that was present before pregnancy or it may arise during pregnancy. Because pregnancy puts special demands on a woman's body, a health problem that is normally under control can change while you are pregnant. Certain medical conditions, such as hypertension and diabetes, should be brought under control before you become pregnant and may require more frequent visits to your doctor or other special attention. Changes in your life style may also be in order, and your doctor may be able to offer suggestions for improving it.

If you've had a problem in a previous pregnancy, that doesn't necessarily mean that the problem will recur or that you shouldn't try again. Some problems develop a pattern of repeating, but most do not. If a problem is apt to be repeated, you should be aware in advance that you may need special attention before and during your pregnancy.

If you have a family history of birth defects, your doctor may suggest that you see a genetic counselor. Genetic counseling can also help identify a pattern of inherited disorders, if one exists. Common genetic disorders and the way they are inherited are reviewed in Chapter 6.

Your preconception visit is a time for you to ask questions, too. Don't hesitate to ask for advice or discuss any concerns you might have. Your doctor is there to provide information and guidance.

Diet and Weight

A balanced diet is a basic part of good health at all times in your life. The foods you eat are the main source of the nutrients for your fetus, the term used to refer to the baby while it is growing inside you during pregnancy. As the fetus grows and places new demands on your body, you will need more of most nutrients than you did in the past. A good prepregnancy diet is the best way to ensure that you and your fetus start out with the nutrients you both need.

Your body functions best when it is well fueled with a balanced diet. To choose that diet, you should be aware of what nutrients your body requires, how much of each nutrient you need, and which foods are good sources. Healthy eating practices are not just for pregnancy, but for the rest of your life. An appropriate healthy diet can easily be modified during pregnancy to provide the extra calories you need. Nutrition in general and the extra needs of pregnancy are discussed in Chapter 8.

Special Diets

Your doctor may detect needs in your diet that should be met before you become pregnant. The factors listed below can affect how your body uses nutrients. If any of these factors apply to you, consult your doctor, because you may need to change your diet.

- Do you take medication (prescription or over-the-counter) regularly?
- Do you follow a strict vegetarian diet?
- Do you run long distances or perform strenuous exercise on a regular basis?
- Do you fast?
- Do you follow a reducing diet?
- Do you have a history of anemia?

Phenylketonuria is an inherited condition that keeps the body from processing an essential amino acid found in foods that contain protein. As a result, the levels of this amino acid build up in the mother's body and can cause birth defects and mental retardation in the fetus. If you were treated for phenylketouria, probably as a child, you still have the disorder, even if there are no signs of it. However, by following a special diet before pregnancy, you can help keep this condition from affecting your baby during pregnancy, even though there is still a small chance that the baby will inherit the disorder. Before trying to become pregnant, you should consult a doctor and be following a special diet if you have phenylketouria.

Weight

Every woman would like to maintain an ideal weight for her height. If you're planning to have a baby, however, it's important that you not be excessively underweight or overweight before pregnancy. Underweight women tend to have smaller babies. This is not an advantage, however, because smaller babies have more problems during labor and in the nursery. In general, being overweight is a health hazard. During pregnancy, being overweight is linked to having high blood pressure or diabetes. Extreme obesity puts a strain on the heart that becomes an added burden during pregnancy. Women who are over-weight are also more prone to discomforts during pregnancy. It is not a good idea to be on a weight-loss diet while you are pregnant or trying to become pregnant, however. This type of diet could deny you and your baby the nutrients you both need. The best way to plan for

Overweight or Overfat?

Fat is the form in which energy is stored. If a diet provides excess calories, they are stored as fat. Obesity is having too much fat. It is difficult to define exactly when a person goes from being slightly fat to being obese. A standard method is to compare a person's body weight with the "ideal" weight for someone who has the same height and frame. If you weigh over 20% more than this weight, you are obese.

Body weight is not always a good measure of the amount of fat you have, though. A person who exercises loses fat and builds up muscle, which is heavier than fat. So a physically fit person can have a body weight that is above normal, but an amount of fat that is below normal. By contrast, a person who is not very active may weigh just as much as a physically fit person, but the inactive person will have more fat and less muscle. Generally, it is normal for a woman to have up to 20–25% of her total body weight in fat.

Height and Weight for Women*

Height		Weight (lb)		
Feet	Inches	Small Frame	Medium Frame	Large Frame
4	9	99–108	106–118	115–128
4	10	100–110	108–120	117–131
4	11	101–112	110–123	119–134
5	0	103–115	112–126	122–137
5	1	105–118	115–129	125–141
5	2	108–121	118–132	128–144
5	3	111–124	121–135	131–148
5	4	114–127	124–138	134–152
5	5	117–130	127–141	137–156
5	6	120–133	130–144	140–160
5	7	123–136	133–147	143–164
5	8	126–139	136–150	146–167
5	9	129–142	139–153	149–170
5	10	132–145	142–156	152–173
5	11	135–148	145–159	155–176

* Height shown is without shoes, and weight is without clothes.

your pregnancy is to try to reach an ideal weight before you become pregnant. You will be more comfortable during pregnancy, and the extra weight you gain will be easier to lose later.

Exercise

Good health at any time in your life depends not only on proper diet but also on getting enough exercise. What you can do in sports and exercise during pregnancy depends on your health and, in part, on how active you are before you become pregnant (for specific guidelines, see Chapter 7).

When beginning a program, decide whether you want to improve your heart and lung function, the tone of your body muscles, or both. Then, select exercises that will enable you to meet your goals. If you are not used to being active, you should begin an exercise program gradually.

Exercises to improve your heart and lung function can be measured by keeping track of your heart rate. When you know how your heart rate responds to exercise, you can find out how hard to exercise.

Your Target Heart Rate

To find your target heart rate, look for the age category closest to your age and read across. For example, if you are 29, the closest age on the chart is 30; the target heart rate is 114–142 beats per minute. Your maximum heart rate is 220 minus your age. Your target heart rate is 60–75% of the maximum. These figures are averages to be used as general guidelines.

Target Heart Rate for Nonpregnant Women*

Age (years)	Target Heart Rate (beats per minute)	Average Maximum Heart Rate (beats per minute)
20	120–150	200
25	117–146	195
30	114–142	190
35	111–138	185
40	108–135	180
45	105–131	175

* National Heart, Lung, and Blood Institute. Exercise and your heart. NIH Publication No. 81-1677. Washington, DC: U.S. Government Printing Office, 1981

You should exercise so that your heart beats at your target heart rate, because this is the level that gives you the best workout.

Every time you exercise, you should begin with a 5- to 10-minute period of light activity, such as brisk walking, as a warm-up before each session. Once your body is warmed up, exercise for 20–30 minutes at your target heart rate. After this 20–30-minute period, you should have a cool-down period of 5–10 minutes. During this period, you gradually reduce your activity, allowing your heart rate to return to a near-normal level.

A program for toning muscles usually requires exercise at least three times a week. It does not have to be done daily—some people's muscles cannot withstand hard exercise every day. Every other day is fine. But it is important that you maintain your routine throughout the year. If you stop for 6–8 weeks, you will need to start again at a lower level of exertion, as if you are just beginning a muscle-toning program.

Cigarettes, Alcohol, and Drugs

Tobacco, alcohol, and drugs are addictive and can harm both you and your fetus. They can have bad effects on the fetus at a time when organs are forming, causing damage that can last a lifetime or even result in death.

Used in combination, as these substances often are, they are even more dangerous. For the sake of your own health and that of your baby, now is a good time to quit or at least cut down your use of tobacco, alcohol, and illegal drugs. By quitting, a pregnant woman helps not only herself, but also her fetus.

It takes time and patience to quit a habit. This is especially true if you've had that habit for a long time. Don't be embarrassed. Ask for help. Your doctor can offer support and medical advice. He or she can also suggest ways to get through the withdrawal stage of quitting. Your decision to quit may be one of the most difficult things you've ever done, but it will be one of the most worthwhile.

Stopping Birth Control

Birth control pills regulate your menstrual cycle. Once you've stopped taking them, your periods may be irregular for a while. This can make it difficult to detect your fertile times, as well as your due date when you become pregnant. Using birth control pills before you become pregnant does not cause any birth defects, regardless of how close to conception you stop using them.

If you have been using an intrauterine device (IUD) to prevent pregnancy, it should be removed before you try to conceive. It is thought that the IUD works by preventing the egg from being fertilized, but pregnancy can occur with an IUD in place. If pregnancy occurs with the IUD in place, it can be harmful; therefore, it should be removed right away by a doctor.

Environment

Some substances found in the environment or at the work place can make it more difficult for a woman to become pregnant or can harm the fetus of a pregnant woman. If you are planning to become pregnant, you may wish to look closely at your work place and environment. If you see that you could be exposed to a harmful substance, then you can take steps to avoid it (see "Harmful Agents," Chapter 7).

Before you accept a job, find out from your employer whether you might be exposed to toxic substances, chemicals, or radiation. Talk to the personnel office about maternity leave, medical benefits, and disability coverage. Once employed, discuss your level of exposure to specific substances with your employee health division, personnel office, or union representative.

Radiation, an invisible form of energy transmitted in waves, is used in some jobs. It is also used to diagnose and treat disease in the form of X-rays. Exposure to high levels of some kinds of radiation can affect the fertility of men and women, as well as affect the fetus of a pregnant woman. Women planning a pregnancy who are exposed to ionizing radiation in industrial and medical settings should ask for monthly readings of the amount of radiation to which they have been exposed. The amount of radiation received in a chest X-ray, for instance, will not hurt fertility or a fetus. When radiation is used to treat disease such as cancer, however, it is used in much larger amounts and can be harmful.

Exposure to chemicals such as lead, certain solvents, or certain insecticides can reduce your partner's fertility by killing or damaging his sperm. Unlike women, who are born with their complete supply of eggs, men produce sperm most of their lives. Unless the damage to a man's reproductive system is very serious, he will probably be able to produce healthy sperm again a short time after his exposure to the dangerous material stops. Some pesticides can also damage a woman's eggs, but not as much is known about the effects of chemicals on eggs.

Vaccination

Infection with measles, mumps, or rubella during pregnancy can cause serious birth defects or illness in the fetus. Some vaccines to prevent these diseases may also be harmful to the fetus. Your doctor may want to ensure your immunity before pregnancy—either by vaccination, documentation of previous exposure, or testing. If you have never had these diseases or do not think you have been vaccinated against them, your doctor may suggest that you be vaccinated before you become pregnant. The vaccine should be given at least 3 months before you try to conceive. During that time you should be using a method of birth control.

If you plan to travel to areas where you may be exposed to infectious diseases not found in this country, you may need to be vaccinated against these diseases. If you are not using birth control, consult your doctor regarding possible effects during pregnancy (see "Travel," Chapter 7, and the "Vaccines" sidebar, Chapter 12).

Sexually Transmitted Diseases

Diseases that are transmitted through sexual contact—sexually transmitted diseases—come in all types and forms. Sexually transmitted diseases not only can affect your ability to conceive but can also infect and harm your baby.

The use of some contraceptive methods, such as condoms and spermicides, can lower the risk of getting a sexually transmitted disease. Couples trying to conceive will not be using these forms of contraception. Therefore, they may be at higher risk of getting a sexually transmitted disease if they have more than one sexual partner.

If you think you may have a sexually transmitted disease, see your doctor right away for the appropriate tests and treatment. Your partner should also be treated, and you both should abstain from any sexual intercourse until you have completed treatment.

Chlamydia, Gonorrhea, and Pelvic Inflammatory Disease

Chlamydial and gonorrheal infections are the most common sexually transmitted diseases in the United States today. It is thought that about 20–40% of all sexually active women have probably been exposed to chlamydia at some time. People who have or have had gonorrhea are more likely to have a chlamydial infection as well, because the two diseases often travel together.

Chlamydial and gonorrheal infections can cause pelvic inflammatory disease, or PID. This is a severe infection that spreads from the vagina and cervix through the pelvic area and may involve the uterus, fallopian tubes, and ovaries. The fallopian tubes, through which an egg travels from the ovary to the uterus, also may become scarred and blocked. If this happens, a woman may not be able to

How Sexually Transmitted Diseases Can Affect You and Your Baby

Disease	Symptoms in Women	Effects On: Mother	Effects On: Fetus/Baby
AIDS	Appetite or weight loss, fatigue, swollen lymph nodes, night sweats, fever or chills, persistent diarrhea or cough	Immune system damage, leading to infections (such as pneumonia) or cancers; death	Immune system damage leading to death in 1–2 years in most infants
Chlamydia	Genital burning or itching, vaginal discharge, painful or frequent urination, pelvic pain; may be no symptoms	Pelvic inflammatory disease, ectopic pregnancy	Eye infection, pneumonia
Gonorrhea	Vaginal discharge, minor genital irritation; most women have no symptoms	Pelvic inflammatory disease, infertility, arthritis	Eye infection if left untreated
Genital herpes	Flu-like symptoms (fever, chills, muscle aches, etc); small, painful, fluid-filled blisters on genitals or buttocks	Recurrent outbreaks	Severe skin infection, nervous system damage, blindness, mental retardation, death
Genital warts	Possible genital itching, irritation, or bleeding; warts may appear as small, cauliflower-shaped clusters	Warts grow in size and number, cancerous changes	Warts may block vaginal opening
Syphilis	A painless open sore called a chancre; later rash, sluggishness, or slight fever	Damage to heart, blood vessels, and nervous system; blindness, insanity, death	Miscarriage, stillbirth, syphilis in liveborn infant

have children. In cases of prolonged or repeated pelvic infection, surgery may be needed to remove damaged reproductive organs.

Gonorrhea and chlamydia can infect the fetus as it passes through the vagina during delivery, causing eye infection and other complications. A newborn's eyes are very sensitive to gonorrhea, and blindness may result. To help prevent this, the eyes of newborns are treated at birth. This is done for every baby whether or not the mother has a history of gonorrhea.

Men with chlamydial and gonorrheal infections commonly have the symptom of a drip from the penis. Many women have no symptoms and find out they have chlamydia or gonorrhea only when their sexual partners are found to have the disease. Sometimes a pelvic exam is not enough to confirm a diagnosis, and other tests may need to be performed. If you have these diseases, you can be treated with drugs that are safe to take during pregnancy.

Herpes Simplex Virus

Genital herpes is an infection caused by herpes simplex virus. It produces sores and blisters on or around the sex organs. It is transmitted during sexual activity through direct contact with a person who has active sores. Some people have only one outbreak; others have repeated bouts. Although it is rare, the baby can become infected with the herpes virus during birth. As a result the baby may suffer severe skin infection, damage to the nervous system, blindness, mental retardation, or death.

If you have ever had genital herpes or have had sexual contact with someone who has, tell your doctor. He or she may want to schedule more frequent examinations and possible testing to diagnose herpes. If there are signs of active infection when you are in labor, your doctor may plan for a cesarean birth. Cesarean birth reduces the chance that the baby will come in contact with the virus in the vagina, because delivery takes place through a surgical cut in the abdomen. When there are no herpes lesions, the baby can be delivered vaginally.

Human Papillomavirus

Human papillomavirus is a virus that causes genital warts (sometimes called condyloma). Warts in the genital area are easily passed from person to person during sexual intercourse and oral and anal sex.

Although some warts may disappear on their own, in most cases treatment is needed. Warts often can be successfully treated during pregnancy. If warts are extensive, though, it may be best to wait until after delivery to begin treatment. In any case, your doctor will want to watch your condition closely throughout your entire pregnancy.

Syphilis

Syphilis remains a dangerous sexually transmitted disease. If untreated, it often spreads throughout the body and can cause blindness, heart disease, nervous disorders, insanity, tumors, and death. Syphilis can be passed from a pregnant woman's bloodstream to her fetus, sometimes causing *miscarriage* or *stillbirth*. If the infant lives, it may be born with congenital syphilis. Infants with congenital syphilis may have problems involving the nervous system, skin, bones, liver, lungs, or spleen.

Syphilis can be very hard to detect in women. The sore or *chancre* that marks the site of infection may be in the vagina where it cannot be seen. For most heterosexual men, the chancre appears on the penis, but it may be anywhere around the genital area.

In its early stages, when a chancre is present, syphilis may be diagnosed by examining the fluid from the chancre. A blood test may or may not find the disease in the earliest stages. The chancre will disappear even without treatment, but the disease remains. After the chancre has disappeared, the only sure method for diagnosing syphilis is a blood test.

Treating an infected pregnant woman will halt further damage to her fetus, but it will not reverse any harm already done. If treatment is completed during the first 3–4 months of pregnancy, it is very unlikely that the infant will suffer any long-term damage. Treating an infected infant after birth will usually prevent further damage but will probably not reverse any damage already done.

HIV Infection and AIDS

Human immune deficiency virus (HIV) infection and acquired immune deficiency syndrome (AIDS), the disease caused by HIV, are growing threats to women. Once in the bloodstream, HIV invades and destroys cells of the immune system, the body's natural defense against disease, leaving it open to harmful infections that can cause death. When a person infected with HIV comes down with one of these serious infections, he or she is said to have AIDS. Once established, the infection persists for life and is nearly always fatal. It may take more than 5 years for symptoms to appear; meanwhile, the virus can spread, both to sexual partners and to a fetus.

The virus is passed from person to person through body fluids: blood, semen (a mixture of sperm and fluid that a man releases during orgasm), and possibly vaginal fluid. The most common ways these fluids are exchanged are through contact with infected blood during intravenous drug use, sexual contact, and to a fetus from its infected mother's blood.

About one-third of the time, the virus is passed to the fetus during pregnancy. Most infected babies die within 3 years after birth. Because the virus can be passed across the *placenta* before birth, it makes no difference whether the baby is born through the vagina or by cesarean delivery—infection may already have occurred. A mother who is breast-feeding may infect her infant after birth because the AIDS virus is present in breast milk. This means that even if a woman remains free of infection during her pregnancy, she could still pass the virus on to her newborn through her breast milk if she were to become infected shortly after delivery.

If you think that you may have been exposed to the AIDS virus, it is important to talk with your doctor about being tested. Research is ongoing, and it may be possible for the condition to be treated.

A test called the enzyme-linked immunosorbent assay (ELISA) is used to detect HIV. It will show whether your blood contains HIV *antibodies*—a sign that you have been infected. Positive results are then confirmed by Western blot, another test used as a double check. If both tests are positive, you are considered to be infected. A positive test does not mean that you have AIDS; it means that you have been infected with HIV and that you run a high risk of getting AIDS and passing it on to others. About 1 time in 20,000, the tests will give a false-positive result. A false-positive result means that the test indicates that you have been infected when you haven't been.

There are other factors that can cause less-than-accurate test results. After exposure to the virus, several weeks to several months are usually required before enough antibodies show up in the blood to produce a positive test result. This means that if you were exposed to the virus only a week before being tested, the test would show a negative result. A negative test can't tell you whether you are now infected; it only indicates that you didn't have antibodies when the test was done. A negative test also doesn't mean that you are immune to AIDS. You still need to protect yourself from infection.

You are at risk of being infected with HIV and getting AIDS if you:

- Use intravenous drugs
- Have sex with someone who has multiple partners, uses intravenous drugs, or is bisexual
- Had a blood transfusion before 1983

To protect yourself, your children, and others, you should change any risk-taking behavior and be tested for the presence of antibodies to the virus in your blood.

Medical Conditions

Some women have medical conditions, such as diabetes (high blood sugar), hypertension (high blood pressure), or cardiovascular (circulatory) problems that will call for special care during pregnancy. These medical problems are more easily managed if they are well under control *before* you become pregnant. This is another reason why talking to your doctor about your pregnancy plans is a good idea. The effects of these conditions during pregnancy are discussed in Chapter 10.

Pregnancy at 35 and Older

If you are in your mid-30s or older and are planning to have a baby, you're not alone. The trend toward delaying parenthood is a growing one. More and more couples are starting their families later in life. In the past decade, the rate at which women in their 30s had their first child almost doubled.

Most women who have children in their 30s or 40s have uncomplicated pregnancies and bear healthy children. Women who want to delay parenthood—or to continue to bear children in their 30s—often have concerns about their ability to become pregnant, the effects on their health, and the health of their baby. Some of these concerns are valid, but others are not. In general, women retain their good health and their ability to have healthy children into their 40s, although becoming pregnant may be more difficult.

Women age physically over time, not all at once. The potential for problems during pregnancy and childbirth does increase slightly each year beyond a woman's early 30s, but there is no age at which there is a sudden dramatic change.

The risk of infant death within the first year of life is almost the same for babies born to mothers 25–29 years of age and to mothers 30–34 years of age. The risk increases slightly in women who have their first babies when they are 35–39, and more significantly once a woman reaches her 40s.

A woman's fertility gradually declines as she reaches her mid-30s. One reason for this is that a woman ovulates—releases an egg for fertilization—less often as she ages. The number of eggs available for fertilization decreases with age, so you may not be ovulating every month, even though you have a menstrual period. You may spend several extra months trying to conceive before becoming pregnant. This wait can be trying if you are eager to become pregnant.

The likelihood of birth defects increases with age, but it remains low well into a woman's 30s. Women 35 and older are usually tested for genetic disorders such as Down syndrome, a disease that is linked to mental retardation and other medical problems. (Down syndrome used to be called mongolism, but this term is no longer used.)

Any of these factors could be a risk, but they do not necessarily mean that you won't have a normal, healthy baby. They do require that you be informed about potential problems and discuss your plans with your doctor to ensure that you get the proper medical attention that any special concerns require.

Questions to Consider...

- Should I gain or lose weight before pregnancy?
- Do I have any special dietary needs?
- Does my use of alcohol, tobacco, or drugs interfere with my chance of having a healthy pregnancy?
- Could any of the over-the-counter medications I'm taking be harmful to my baby?
- Should I start an exercise program? Can I continue my present exercise program?
- Does my work expose me to things that could be harmful during pregnancy?
- Do I need to be vaccinated for any infectious diseases before I try to conceive?
- Should I be tested for any sexually transmitted diseases?

Chapter 2

How Reproduction Occurs

A general understanding of the reproductive process, particularly fertilization and ovulation, will help as you prepare for pregnancy. Knowing how your body works will help you identify the time in your menstrual cycle when you are most fertile.

The Menstrual Cycle

A woman's fertility revolves around her menstrual cycle. Each month her ovaries produce an egg. The uterus is prepared for pregnancy by development of a thick lining in which the egg will grow if it is fertilized. If the egg isn't fertilized, the lining is shed during the menstrual period and the cycle begins again.

The changes that take place in the menstrual cycle are caused by hormones—substances normally produced by the body to control certain functions:

- *Follicle-stimulating hormone (FSH)* and *luteinizing hormone (LH)* are produced by the *pituitary gland* (a small organ located at the base of the brain) and cause eggs to mature and be released.
- *Estrogen* and *progesterone* are produced by the ovaries and prepare the lining of the uterus to nourish a fertilized egg.
- *Human chorionic gonadotropin (hCG)* is produced by cells that eventually form the *placenta* once the fertilized egg has developed and attached to the uterine wall.

Days 1–5 of the menstrual cycle are called menstruation, during which the endometrium (lining of the uterus) breaks down and is shed through the vagina during your monthly menstrual period. This shedding is triggered by a drop in the levels of the hormones estrogen and progesterone, which occurs when an egg is not fertilized.

The drop in estrogen and progesterone signals the pituitary to send a surge of the hormone FSH to the ovaries. During days 1–13 of the menstrual cycle, FSH stimulates follicles in the ovaries to produce estrogen. Follicles are structures that produce the egg inside the ovary. Each month one follicle is the source of the egg for that cycle. The estrogen made by the follicle causes the endometrium to begin to thicken and develop. Cervical mucus becomes thinner and clearer during this phase.

Ovulation

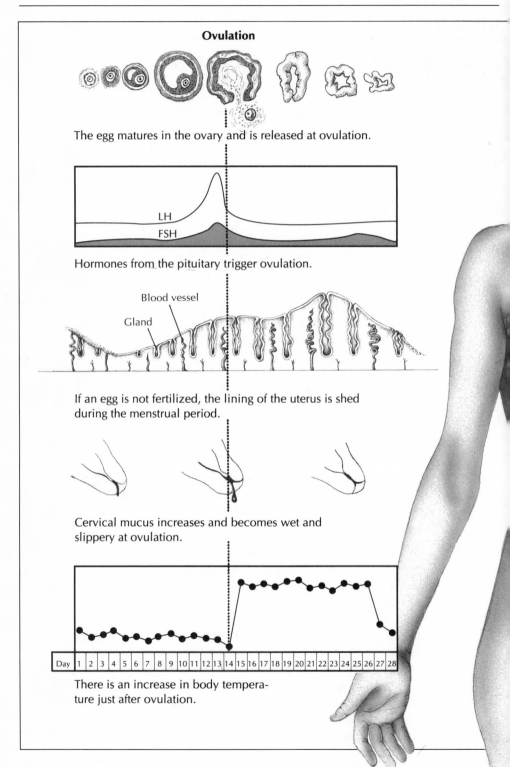

The egg matures in the ovary and is released at ovulation.

Hormones from the pituitary trigger ovulation.

If an egg is not fertilized, the lining of the uterus is shed during the menstrual period.

Cervical mucus increases and becomes wet and slippery at ovulation.

There is an increase in body temperature just after ovulation.

Pituitary gland

The pituitary gland triggers the release of hormones that cause an egg to mature and be released at ovulation during a woman's monthly cycle.

4

1

3

2

Ovary

Ovaries

Uterus

The Growth of an Egg

The egg matures in the follicle *(1)* and is released at ovulation *(2)*. The follicle develops into the corpus luteum *(3)*, which shrinks and disappears if pregnancy does not occur *(4)*.

Ovulation—the release of an egg from one of the ovaries—occurs on day 14 in the average 28-day cycle. The increased amount of estrogen produced by the follicles, in addition to stimulating the endometrium, also causes an increase in LH, which in turn triggers the follicle to release the egg. Once the egg is released, it can be fertilized for 12–24 hours.

After ovulation, the follicle is changed into the corpus luteum. During the second half of the cycle, the corpus luteum produces progesterone, which causes further thickening of the lining of the uterus.

When fertilization does not occur, estrogen and progesterone production drops sharply. This drop triggers the endometrium to shed, marking the beginning of another menstrual cycle.

The average menstrual cycle lasts 28 days but may range from 23–35 days. The time frames given here for the various phases of the menstrual cycle are only averages. Your own cycle will probably vary somewhat from month to month. It's a good idea to keep a diary of your menstrual cycle so you will know what is normal for you.

If fertilization does occur, the developing placenta, which nourishes the fetus in the uterus, produces the hormone hCG. This is the hormone measured in pregnancy tests. During the early stages of pregnancy, hCG stimulates the follicle that has released the egg (the corpus luteum) to produce estrogen and progesterone. The increase in estrogen and progesterone that occurs during pregnancy prevents ovulation and menstruation during pregnancy.

Ovulation—
Fertilization—Implantation
The egg is released from the ovary at
ovulation (1), *is fertilized by sperm in the*
fallopian tube (2), *and moves through the*
tube to the lining of the uterus (3), *where*
it becomes implanted and grows.

Ovary
Uterus
Fallopian tube
Cervix
Vagina

Detecting Ovulation

Women who wish to plan when they become pregnant can do so by timing intercourse near the time they ovulate. There are several ways to detect ovulation. One way is by monitoring your basal body temperature. A woman using this method takes her temperature every morning before getting out of bed and records it on a graph. Most women have a slight but detectable rise in their normal body temperature after ovulation. This method is useful in showing a pattern you can use to predict when you will ovulate in future cycles. It cannot be used to predict ovulation in the month in which the temperature is recorded, because your temperature pattern is not complete until the month is over, and because your temperature does not begin to go up until ovulation has already occurred.

Another way to detect ovulation is by observing changes in the amount and makeup of the fluid, called cervical mucus, that normally is released from the vagina. Women who use this method learn to recognize the changes that occur in cervical mucus around the time of ovulation. The fertile period starts with the first signs of mucus and continues through the peak day.

Kits that will help detect ovulation can be purchased in a drugstore without a prescription. These kits contain chemicals that show the LH surge that comes just before ovulation. They must be used exactly according to instructions.

Fertilization

About every 28 days an egg is released from one of the ovaries into the nearby fallopian tube. Once the egg is in the tube, it moves slowly toward the uterus. If a man's sperm does not fertilize the egg while it is in the tube, the egg continues down the tube to the uterus and is absorbed by the body.

Sperm cells are made in a man's testes, located in the scrotal sac below the penis. When the sperm cells mature, they leave the testes through small tubes called the vas deferens. These tubes carry the sperm to a larger tube in the penis called the urethra. As sperm travel from the testes, they mix with fluid from the seminal vesicles and prostate gland (a gland that produces most of the fluid for ejaculation). This mixture of sperm and fluid is called semen. When the man ejaculates or climaxes during intercourse, semen travels through the urethra in the penis into the vagina. It is not necessary for a woman to climax to become pregnant.

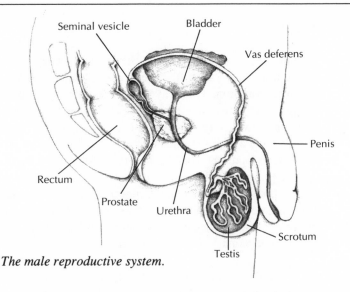

The male reproductive system.

        Pregnancy can occur if you have sexual intercourse during or
near the time of ovulation. When the man ejaculates, his sperm are
released into the vagina. They then travel up through the cervix, into
the uterus, and out into the fallopian tubes. If live sperm meet a ripe
egg in one of the tubes, fertilization can occur. The ripe egg can
survive only about 12–24 hours, but sperm normally can live 2–3 days
or longer. The fertilized egg then moves through the tube into the
uterus and becomes attached there to grow and develop.

Infertility

        Many couples who want a child face the problem of infertility—they
have tried to conceive but have not been able to do so. Couples are
considered infertile if they have not been able to conceive after 1 year
of regular sexual intercourse without the use of any form of birth
control. Infertility occurs in about 15% of all couples. If you don't
get pregnant after trying for 6–12 months, you may wish to explore
special tests and techniques.

The Infertility Evaluation

        Couples who are infertile and want to conceive a child should think
about having a complete infertility evaluation. Usually examinations
for infertility begin with a medical history and general physical
examination of the man and the woman. A medical history of the

woman includes questions about any past illnesses, such as appendicitis or pelvic infections, that might have damaged her reproductive organs.

The couple will also be asked about their sexual relations to find out whether their infertility may be related to such factors as timing or frequency of intercourse. Often a couple may simply need more information on the sexual techniques that are most favorable to conception. Timing sexual intercourse to take place just before ovulation, for example, increases the chances of conception.

These initial examinations are then followed by more extensive testing of both the man and the woman to detect the exact cause of the infertility and to find out whether it can be treated. Depending on the cause of the infertility, alternatives are available.

Alternatives

If a woman is fertile and her partner is infertile, artificial insemination may be an option. For this procedure, semen is obtained from a donor who has been carefully screened for characteristics chosen by the couple. This screening also ensures that the donor does not have any serious diseases that could be transmitted to the woman. This semen, and the sperm it contains, is inseminated, or introduced, into the woman's vagina. At present, frozen instead of fresh semen is generally used.

If a woman is infertile because of blocked fallopian tubes, she may have surgery to open them. If surgery doesn't work, pregnancy may be possible with a procedure called *in vitro fertilization (IVF)*. It involves inducing ovulation with medications that cause multiple eggs to be produced. These eggs are removed from the ovary with the aid of a laparoscope or ultrasound. They are then fertilized with the man's sperm in a dish in the laboratory. The fertilized eggs are then transferred back into the mother's uterus through her vagina.

A variation of this technique is *gamete intrafallopian transfer (GIFT)*. It is considered closer to normal fertilization than IVF because the egg and sperm are joined inside the woman's body instead of in a laboratory dish. After the egg and the sperm are obtained as for IVF, they are both put in the woman's fallopian tube, where the egg is fertilized.

These methods are new and may not be widely used in your area. They also involve special considerations that must be carefully weighed by a couple and their doctor. Such alternatives are not for everyone and usually are considered when other methods don't work.

Questions to Consider...

- How can I tell when I have ovulated?
- If I'm trying to conceive, when it the best time to have intercourse?
- What would be the best way to keep a record of my menstrual periods?
- Do I need an infertility workup?

Section II

Pregnancy

Section II

Pregnancy

Pregnancy is a time of tremendous change. From the very beginning, your baby-to-be brings about major changes not only in your body but also in your daily life. For 9 months, the fetus is totally dependent on you for its nutrients and its life functions. One of the most important things you can do for your baby is to be responsible for a healthy life style and for getting early and regular prenatal care.

Most babies are born healthy. A small number of women, however, develop problems with their pregnancies. Complications can arise at any time during pregnancy, sometimes without warning. If you are receiving regular care, your doctor may be able to detect signs that you may need special attention.

Advances in medicine have helped both to decrease the risk of childbirth and to improve the health of babies at birth. But there are no guarantees of a perfect outcome. By receiving early and regular prenatal care, making carefully thought-out decisions, and having a healthy life style, you become a truly active participant in your pregnancy and can be assured that you're doing everything you can to have a healthy baby.

Chapter 3

A New Life Begins

After the sperm from the man enters and fertilizes the woman's egg in the fallopian tube, the fertilized egg becomes implanted in the wall of the uterus. The developing baby is called an embryo for the first 8 weeks after fertilization. After that it is known as a fetus. For all 40 weeks of pregnancy, the cells of the fetus grow and multiply at an incredible rate—from that first single cell that carries the "blueprint" for the baby's entire physical development to a completely formed individual weighing on the average about 7 pounds and measuring about 20 inches in length.

Early Signs of Pregnancy

The sign that most women associate with pregnancy is a missed menstrual period. But not all women have regular periods. Menstrual periods can be affected by stress or illnesses, so it is best to watch for a number of other signs:

- Scanty menstrual period or spotting
- Breast tenderness
- Extreme tiredness
- Nausea
- Bloated sensation
- Frequent urination

If you have one or more of these symptoms along with a missed period, you should consider that you may be pregnant, even if you have been using birth control.

Diagnosis of Pregnancy

It used to be necessary to wait until you missed two periods to have a pregnancy test. Today pregnancy can be confirmed about a week after you miss a period. During early pregnancy, the hormone called *human chorionic gonadotropin (hCG)*, which is produced by the developing *placenta*, is present in the mother's urine and blood. You can take a urine sample to your doctor or to a clinic, or you can test it yourself with a home pregnancy test kit. If the test shows that you are

31

pregnant, you should make an appointment with your doctor to confirm the pregnancy and begin prenatal care.

There are many home pregnancy test kits that you can buy without a prescription. All of the tests check for the presence of hCG in your urine. If your body has produced enough hCG, a chemical in the test kit will react with the hCG that is in your urine. The tests show the presence of the hCG in different ways. In some, a ring forms in a liquid or a bead changes color.

In general, the tests require that you use a sample of the first urine you pass in the morning. It has the highest amount of hCG in it. Don't use the urine if it is cloudy or discolored. A small part of the urine will be added to a powder or liquid in the test kit. With some kits, the urine is mixed with the test solution and then left to sit for a certain amount of time. Other kits have more steps to follow, and you may need to time each of the steps accurately. The amount of time needed to get a result can vary, but often a result is available within an hour.

The test can easily give a wrong result if the directions are not followed. Be sure to follow the directions of the test exactly:

• Use only clean containers—never reuse the containers in the kit.
• Time the test for the exact number of minutes required.
• Leave the test in a place away from heat and where it will not be bumped.

A few medical conditions or some drugs can cause the test to turn out positive even if you aren't pregnant. A negative test may mean either that you are not pregnant or that you are pregnant but your body hasn't made enough hCG yet to be detected by the test. Many kits contain two complete tests so that you can test your urine again in a few days if the first test is negative.

Home pregnancy tests can be very accurate, but no test is 100% foolproof. False-negative results (showing you are not pregnant when you really are) can occur in a small number of cases. A blood test for pregnancy, performed in a laboratory, is more accurate. With home testing, a negative result—showing that you are not pregnant—should not be considered foolproof. The results of a home pregnancy test, whether positive or negative, should be confirmed by your doctor as soon as possible.

Growth and Development

During pregnancy the fetus grows in the mother's uterus. As described in Chapter 2, the uterus is located in the pelvic cavity between the bladder and the rectum. Almost as soon as pregnancy occurs, the lining of the uterus begins to thicken and its blood vessels enlarge in order to nourish the growing fetus. The uterus changes continually throughout pregnancy, expanding as the fetus grows.

The placenta begins to form and grow as soon as the fertilized egg attaches to the lining of the uterus. Also known as the afterbirth, the placenta is the channel through which oxygen, nutrients, drugs, hormones, and other substances pass from mother to fetus. In the opposite direction, waste products from the fetus cross through the placenta to the mother via the fetal vessels of the umbilical cord to be disposed of by her body.

The placenta starts as small sprouts growing from the wall of the fertilized egg. In these sprouts, called *chorionic villi,* fetal blood vessels form. The tips of the vessels enter the wall of the uterus and tap the mother's blood vessels. Although the maternal and fetal blood systems are in close contact, the two bloodstreams do not mix. The placenta is expelled from the uterus soon after birth.

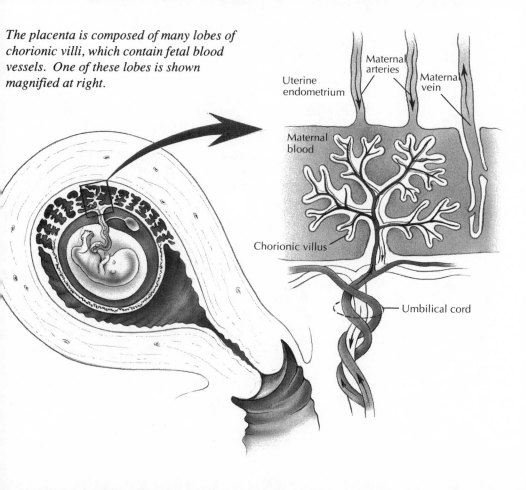

The placenta is composed of many lobes of chorionic villi, which contain fetal blood vessels. One of these lobes is shown magnified at right.

Uterine endometrium

Maternal arteries

Maternal vein

Maternal blood

Chorionic villus

Umbilical cord

Pregnancy Month by Month

The embryo develops rapidly during the first 8 weeks of pregnancy. (Photos courtesy of Carnegie Institution of Washington.)

FETUS

1 st month: By the end of the first month, the embryo has a head and a trunk. Features are beginning to form, and tiny structures called limb buds, which will grow into arms and legs, begin to appear. The heart also forms and begins to beat on the 25th day. At the end of this month, the embryo is about 1/2 inch long and weighs less than 1 ounce.

2 nd month: The early stages of the placenta, chorionic villi, are visible and working. All of the major body organs and systems are formed, although they are not completely developed. The heartbeat can be detected with special techniques. The first bone cells have appeared. Ears, ankles, and wrists are formed, and fingers and toes are developed. Eyelids form and grow but are sealed shut. At the end of the second month, the fetus is a little over 1 inch long but still weighs less than 1 ounce.

3 rd month: Fingers and toes of the fetus have soft nails. There are 20 buds for future teeth, and hair is beginning to appear on the fetus's head. Kidneys develop and secrete urine into the bladder. The initial stages of all organs can be recognized. From now on, the organs will mature and the fetus will gain weight. By the end of this month, the fetus is 4 inches long and weighs a fraction over 1 ounce.

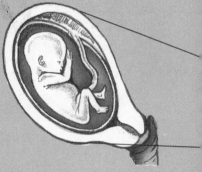

MOTHER

1 *st month:* You may not notice anything different, but your body is going through many changes. The lining of the uterus is thickening. The hormones ***progesterone*** and ***estrogen*** are being produced in increasing quantities. Perhaps you have not had a period (a condition called ***amenorrhea***), or this month's period was very different from normal ones (scanty bleeding or spotting). Your breasts are slightly enlarged and tender, and your nipples may have become more prominent. You probably need to urinate more often, but this will ease in midpregnancy.

2 *nd month:* The total volume of blood in your body increases to accommodate the growing fetus. Your breasts are still tender. You may still be having some of the early discomforts of pregnancy (described in "Physical Changes," Chapter 9) as your body continues to adjust.

3 *rd month:* As you gain weight, your waistline begins to disappear. You may need to start looking for a larger bra and maternity clothes.

Pregnancy Month by Month

FETUS

4 *th month:* The fetus moves, kicks, sleeps and wakes, swallows, can hear, and can pass urine. Eyebrows have formed, and there is a small amount of hair on the head. The skin is pink and transparent. The fetus is now 6–7 inches long and weighs about 5 ounces.

5 *th month:* The fetus has a real growth spurt. The internal organs are maturing. Fingernails have grown to the tips of the fingers. The fetus sleeps and wakes at regular intervals and is much more active, turning from side to side and sometimes moving head over heels. At the end of the month, the fetus is 8–12 inches long and weighs anywhere from 1/2 to 1 pound.

6 *th month:* The fetus is continuing its rapid growth, but its organ systems are still developing. The skin is wrinkled and red and covered with fine, soft hair. At the end of the sixth month, the fetus will be 11–14 inches long and weigh about 1 to 11/2 pounds. But because it is still so small and its lungs are not fully developed, it usually cannot live outside the mother without very specialized care.

MOTHER

4 **th month:** Your abdomen begins to swell with the increased size of the fetus this month. Your nipples and the area around them start to darken. A line running from your navel to your pubic hair may darken (***linea nigra;*** see Chapter 9). Especially if you have dark hair and fair skin, the skin on your face may darken. This condition is called ***chloasma*** and can be brought on or worsened by being in the sun (see "Physical Changes," Chapter 9). The next few months are usually some of the easiest in pregnancy, because most of the early discomforts have disappeared. Sometimes from the end of this month on, you may begin to feel the movement of the fetus. This is called ***quickening*** and feels like a fluttering of wings or like small bubbles. Let your doctor know when you first feel this, because it helps to establish or confirm your due date.

5 **th month:** This month your uterus has expanded to reach the height of your navel, and the skin of the abdomen stretches. If you have not already, you will begin to feel the fetal movements.

6 **th month:** This is your period of greatest weight gain. You may feel the fetus kicking. You may also experience a stitch-like pain at times down the side of your abdomen as the uterine muscle stretches.

Pregnancy Month by Month

FETUS

7th month: This is another rapid growth period for the fetus. It exercises by kicking and stretching. It sucks its thumb and opens and closes its eyes. Calcium is being stored, and fetal bones are hardening. The fetus now has a better chance of survival if it is born early. It is gaining weight—now weighing about 3 pounds—and is about 15 inches long.

8th month: The fetus continues to grow in size and weight. It is too big to move around much, but its kicks are felt much more strongly, and the shape of a small heel or elbow may be visible to you through your abdomen. The bones of the head are soft and flexible. It is now about 18 inches long and weighs about 5 pounds.

9th month: The fetus is now gaining about 1/2 pound per week. The bones of its head are soft and flexible for delivery. It is getting ready for birth and usually settles into a favorable position. It is curled up with its knees against its nose and its thighs tight against its torso, resting lower in the abdomen. At 40 weeks, it will be full term and weigh 6–9 pounds. Your baby should arrive anywhere from 37–42 weeks of pregnancy.

MOTHER

7 *th month:* Increased growth of the fetus adds stress to your system, causing some discomfort. The breasts and uterus continue to increase in size. For some women, stretch marks may appear on the abdomen and breasts, and you may feel ***Braxton–Hicks contractions***, false labor pains.

8 *th month:* Stronger contractions may be felt this month, and you may notice a leakage of ***colostrum***, a fluid secreted from your breasts at the beginning of milk production. Aches and pains due to increased weight may now occur more frequently. Your uterus has grown so that the top part lies just under your diaphragm.

9 *th month:* You may now notice your navel protruding and shortness of breath. Toward the end of this month, when the baby drops into a lower position, you may be able to breathe easier and may have an increased need to urinate. Your cervix will soften, and contractions will increase. Colostrum leakage may be increasing. Discomforts caused by the pressure and weight of the fetus are common, and you often need to rest during the day. Your ankles may swell some at the end of the day.

The growth and development of a fetus has a dramatic effect on a pregnant woman. Although most women experience some of the same physical changes, other changes may be unique to each woman. No two pregnancies are alike. Even for the same woman, a second or third pregnancy may be very different from the first. Understanding the changes that take place in your body and in the growing fetus during pregnancy will help you prepare for the weeks and months to come. Pregnancy usually lasts 280 days, 40 weeks, or about 9 calendar months (of approximately 41/2 weeks each) from the beginning of a woman's last normal menstrual period.

Questions to Consider...

- Did I perform my home pregnancy test correctly?
- Are my early signs of pregnancy normal?
- Now that I'm pregnant, how do I start a program of prenatal care?

Chapter 4

Decisions, Decisions

Pregnant women have many options and choices. They range from
how to prepare for childbirth to where you want the baby to be
delivered and by whom. These important decisions will affect how
comfortable you will be with your care. Thinking now about some of
the decisions and working through them with your partner and your
doctor will help you feel more confident and in control as you approach the birth of your baby. Knowing in advance where and by
whom your baby will be delivered, preparing for the birth with
childbirth classes, and exploring your options regarding breast-feeding
and other aspects of your care will help you make decisions later.

Choosing a Doctor

Choosing who will care for you during your pregnancy and delivery
may be one of your first decisions. Ideally, you have already
chosen your doctor before pregnancy
and have had a chance to discuss

preconception issues. Some women decide on a hospital where they would like to deliver their baby and ask for a referral to a doctor who practices there.

Babies can be delivered by certified nurse–midwives, doctors in family practice, or obstetrician–gynecologists. Certified nurse–midwives are registered nurses specially educated to provide health care to women and their babies from early pregnancy through labor, delivery, and the period after birth. In most states, nurse–midwives must practice with a doctor. They refer patients to a doctor if problems occur. Doctors in family practice provide general care for most conditions, including pregnancy.

Obstetrician–gynecologists are doctors who specialize in the care of women. Most have gone through a 4-year course of specialized training called residency, after graduating from medical school, and have been certified by the American Board of Obstetrics and Gynecology. To be certified, a physician must complete a residency, and then pass a written and oral examination to show that he or she has obtained the special knowledge and skills required for the medical and surgical care of the female reproductive system and related disorders.

If an obstetrician–gynecologist is certified, he or she is eligible to become a Fellow in the American College of Obstetricians and Gynecologists (ACOG), the organization that represents the specialty on both a national and a local level in women's health care issues. ACOG offers a wide variety of continuing medical education programs to help physicians stay current with the latest scientific and clinical practice advances. The initials FACOG behind a doctor's name signify that he or she is a Fellow who specializes in women's health care. A Junior Fellow of ACOG who is in practice has completed a residency program and is preparing to undergo final certification as a specialist in obstetrics and gynecology.

Board-certified obstetricians may become further specialized. One of these subspecialty areas is maternal–fetal medicine. These doctors have additional special training and experience in caring for women whose pregnancies are complicated by medical or obstetric problems. These specialists usually see patients by referral from another doctor.

Many women like to visit doctors and interview them before making a final decision. Feel free to raise questions about other areas of concern to you or your partner. A number of points could affect your choice of a doctor:

- Is the doctor's practice convenient to your home or work?
- Where does the doctor have hospital privileges?

- How do you obtain emergency care outside normal office hours?
- Do you have any problems that may require special care?
- What are the doctor's fees, and how are they covered by your medical insurance plan, if you have one? If you need advice on insurance or a payment plan, the doctor's staff may be able to help.
- Does your insurance plan limit your choice to certain physicians?
- What is the doctor's attitude about questions of concern to you, such as breast-feeding, pain relief, presence of fathers in labor and delivery rooms, and use of birthing rooms?

Another factor to consider is whether the doctor is in a group, collaborative, or solo practice. In a group practice, constant coverage is provided by two or more doctors. You may have a primary doctor and receive care from the others on occasion. It is possible that one of the other members may deliver your baby. This also holds true for collaborative practice, in which a doctor and a nurse or certified nurse–midwife work as a team to provide care before, during, and after pregnancy. With a solo practice, one doctor provides complete care for all of his or her patients. In the event of illness or vacation, coverage is provided by another doctor, whom you may meet in advance.

Both types of practices have advantages and disadvantages. The solo practice allows you to see the same doctor each time, but could involve interruptions, such as canceled appointments when babies arrive unexpectedly, as they often do. The group and collaborative practices have the efficiency of shared resources, but you will receive care from more than one care provider.

The Health Care Team

Many doctors coordinate a team of health care professionals to provide various types of care based on a woman's special needs during pregnancy. The team is made up of persons who will assist your doctor, as well as those who may serve as consultants. The following members may be on the health care team:

- Nurses, who assist obstetricians by providing information needed to diagnose medical conditions, patient education, counseling, and advice on pregnancy nutrition and care
- Childbirth educators, who teach prospective parents about conception, pregnancy, childbirth, and family life

- Certified nurse–midwives, nurses who are specially trained to provide care to women during pregnancy and birth
- Labor and delivery nurses, who help the doctor care for patients in labor and who provide immediate care for babies after birth
- Postpartum nurses, who help care for the mother after birth
- Neonatal nurses, who help care for the newborn
- Dietician or nutritionist, who provides advice and guidance on diet and nutrition and any special needs
- Social workers, who can provide counseling and information about community services for families
- Residents, who are doctors in training at a teaching hospital

During your pregnancy and delivery, your doctor may consult other specialists, who then become a part of the health care team:

- Maternal–fetal medicine subspecialist, to give advice if complications or problems arise
- Geneticist, to detect or manage any inherited disorders or provide counseling on whether such a risk exists
- Neonatologist or pediatrician, to provide special care for the newborn
- Anesthesiologist (a specially trained doctor) to give anesthesia

The health care team can aid your doctor in gathering important information about your pregnancy. This information is used to determine how best to manage your prenatal care and to assess special needs during labor and delivery.

The Setting

The areas for labor and delivery vary from one hospital to another. Your doctor will be able to give you information about the options available.

Many hospitals have responded to the desires of parents-to-be by offering birthing rooms where the family can participate. These rooms may be located in the hospital or nearby. Birthing rooms share the specialized staff and services of a more traditional labor and delivery suite, which may be needed if a problem occurs. They provide a comfortable setting for labor, delivery, and, usually, postpartum recovery. Some allow the mother to remain in the same room for the postpartum stay, so the entire birth process can take place in one room, often with family members present. These rooms are referred to as LDRs (labor/delivery/recovery) or LDRPs (labor/delivery/recovery/postpartum).

There are also freestanding alternative birthing centers that are not in or near a hospital. These centers may not offer all the services that may be needed if an emergency arises. Because of these limitations, a hospital is considered the safest place to give birth.

When selecting your care, you may wish to ask about policies regarding fathers or others in the delivery room. Most hospitals permit support persons to be present in both labor and delivery rooms. It is wise to know the hospital's policy in advance so you can plan accordingly.

Your Childbirth Partner

One of your early decisions will be selecting your childbirth partner to help you through pregnancy, labor, and delivery. Support by a partner from the beginning can ease a woman's pregnancy and help the course of labor and delivery go more smoothly. This person may accompany you on prenatal care visits to your doctor and will attend childbirth preparation classes to assist you in breathing and relaxation exercises. During labor, your partner will take an active role as a coach, helping you carry out what you learned and practiced in childbirth class.

The father of the baby is usually, but not necessarily, the partner. If for some reason the father is not involved in the pregnancy, there are others who can give support and participate actively. A support person can be any family member or friend who will help you and be there for you.

The concept of family-centered care, now widely embraced in modern obstetric practice, focuses on the physical, social, and psychologic needs of the family unit, regardless of the members who may make up that unit. Family-centered care can extend to family members and loved ones who wish to take part in the process.

Childbirth Preparation

Pain or discomfort is a natural part of childbirth for most women. Most pregnant women are concerned about how they will cope with labor and childbirth. It is difficult to know in advance how much pain or discomfort you will have during birth or how you will deal with it. You may find it helpful to learn how pain can be relieved with childbirth preparation techniques or drugs, or a combination of both.

Childbirth preparation is a means of coping with pain and reducing discomfort. The most common methods of preparation—Lamaze, Bradley, and Read—are based on the theory that much of the pain of childbirth is caused by fear and tension. Although there are differences in specific techniques, classes usually seek to relieve pain through the general principles of education, support, relaxation, paced breathing, focusing, and touch.

If you want further information about a particular method of childbirth preparation, ask your doctor to refer you to a childbirth educator. Your doctor can also discuss with you the other types of pain relief that are available (see "Pain Relief," Chapter 13).

Options

Certain decisions, such as those involving breast-feeding, circumcision, sterilization, and selecting an infant car safety seat for the trip home, won't be implemented until after delivery; but they should be thought about in advance. Other issues that may come up during pregnancy that would benefit from preplanning include work and travel considerations, discussed in Chapter 7.

Breast-feeding

One of the most basic decisions you will have to make about the care of your infant is how to feed him or her—with breast milk or formula. During pregnancy, your body prepares to make milk whether or not you plan to breast-feed. Breast milk, including the *colostrum* that appears in the first 2–4 days, is designed by nature to nourish and protect newborns. Infants who are breast-fed have fewer feeding problems, tend to be less constipated, and have fewer infections and allergies.

Others may help you in your decision. Find out your partner's feelings. Ask your doctor, nurse, or childbirth educator any questions you may have. Talk with women who know—some who have breast-fed their babies and others who have decided against it. Your best choice will be the one with which you feel most comfortable. (For further information on breast-feeding, see Chapter 15.)

Circumcision

Parents-to-be often have many questions about circumcision. A man or boy who has not been circumcised has a layer of skin (the foreskin) that covers most of the sensitive end of the penis. Circumcision involves cutting away this skin at the end of the penis. When circumcision is requested by the parents, it is usually done before the baby leaves the hospital.

There is controversy about the need for circumcision. Although it is fairly common in the United States, it is much less common in most other parts of the world. Some parents choose to have their sons circumcised for religious or cultural reasons. There are no laws or hospital rules that require circumcision, however. It is an elective procedure and should be the parents' informed choice. Further information about the procedure is included in Chapter 14.

Sterilization

Couples who decide that they do not want any more children may consider sterilization of either the man or the woman. Almost half of the women who choose sterilization have it done postpartum. It is often performed within a day after delivery, while the woman is still in the hospital.

Because sterilization is permanent, it is a decision that requires careful thought by you and your partner. It is not a decision to make at times of stress or near the end of pregnancy. Therefore, it is appropriate to consider this option as early in pregnancy as possible in order to plan in advance.

If you want to limit the size of your family, you may wish to wait until the health of your newborn is assured before making the decision to be sterilized. For further details about sterilization and other forms of family planning, see Chapter 15.

Infant Safety Seat

Make plans now to bring your infant home in a special infant safety seat. Some states have passed laws requiring the use of infant seats under penalty of fine, and many hospitals will not allow the baby to be

*Be sure to have a car
safety seat that is designed
for a newborn when you
leave the hospital.*

discharged without one. A plastic infant carrier is not a safety seat,
even if a seat belt is placed around it. It can shatter in an accident.
There are various models of infant car seats that are specially designed
to protect babies and small children from harm should a crash occur.
The seats can be rented or purchased. Check with your doctor,
hospital, car dealer, baby stores, or local consumer safety council
about purchase or rental.

Questions to Consider...

- Who are the members of my health care team?
- What options are available in my community in choosing a
  hospital?
- Where can I enroll in a childbirth preparation class?
- Where can I obtain further information on breast-feeding, circumci-
  sion, and sterilization?
- How do I select an infant safety seat?

Chapter 5

Prenatal Care

A program of prenatal care allows your doctor to monitor your health and that of your fetus throughout pregnancy. Although most pregnancies proceed normally, every pregnancy poses some degree of risk. Assessing the risk on an ongoing basis is a central part of prenatal care. At each visit, your doctor will examine you and chart the course of your pregnancy. New techniques provide exciting opportunities to study the fetus. Some of these techniques can help alert your doctor to potential problems.

Even if you previously had a problem-free pregnancy, you should still see your doctor early. No two pregnancies are alike, and complications can arise without warning. Some women who think they are pregnant may delay prenatal care because they are uncertain about continuing the pregnancy. Seeing your doctor can give you the information you may need to make this decision. Your doctor can provide referrals to other counselors, should you need such services in deciding how to manage your pregnancy.

Prenatal care is not just medical care. It also includes childbirth education, counseling, and support of the family. Your doctor can direct you to these services, and you can do your part by participating actively in them.

Regular visits to your doctor are central to your prenatal care. Your first prenatal visit will be longer and more involved than other visits. It will include a history of your health, laboratory tests, a physical examination, and confirmation of the estimated date of delivery—your due date. A schedule will then be set up for subsequent visits and any special tests or instructions you may need. Throughout the process, you should discuss all facets of care with your doctor, and you should feel free to raise questions.

Informed Consent

The process by which you learn what a medical procedure, test, or treatment involves before you grant permission for it is called informed consent. The informed-consent process begins in your doctor's office with a discussion of what you might expect and covers most aspects of your care as described in this book. It is important that you understand this information. Don't be afraid to ask questions or to have your doctor go over anything that isn't clear to you. The physician will note in your record that treatment and risks have been explained to you, and he or she will document your treatment decisions.

As partners in your medical care, both you and your doctor have rights and responsibilities. You have the right to:

- Quality care without discrimination
- Privacy
- Knowledge of the professional status of your care providers and their fees
- Be advised of your diagnosis, treatment, options, and the expected outcome
- Be given an opportunity to be an informed participant
- Refuse treatment
- Participate or refuse to participate in research or any experimentation that affects your care or treatment

You have the responsibility to:

- Provide your doctor with accurate and complete health information
- Let your doctor know that you understand the medical procedures and what you are expected to do

If you do not follow your doctor's plan, or if you refuse treatment, you must accept responsibility for your actions. Your doctor has the right to stop treating you as long as you have time to find another physician. While you are in his or her care, your doctor is responsible for providing you with the best care available.

History

One of the first things you will be asked to provide is information about your health, your family's health, and any past pregnancies. This information can be very helpful in detecting future problems. You are the only one who can provide this information, so it is important that your answers be honest, complete, and accurate. The information is kept private. This information is obtained during preconception care (see the preconceptional care inventory in Chapter 1). If it was not, you will be asked to provide specific information about yourself, the baby's father, and your close family.

The medical history covers your general health. This includes whether you are taking any medications, have any allergies, have any medical conditions, or have been exposed to infections. It also covers your menstrual history, including your last menstrual period, and use

of contraception. Information about habits that may place you at risk
for problems during pregnancy, such as use of alcohol, drugs, or
cigarettes and exposure to harmful agents, should also be provided.

The history of past pregnancies includes details about all former
pregnancies and focuses on problems that may recur: the baby's
weight at birth, how long labor lasted, method of delivery, any complications, or preterm labor. You will be asked to provide information
about pregnancies that you may not have carried to full term.

The family history provides information about any genetic
disorders that may be inherited. If you had a previous child with an
inherited disease, genetic counseling and further studies may be
needed. Your ethnic origin and general life style will also be covered
to determine whether there are any factors that might affect your
health or that of your baby. Chapter 6 includes further details about
genetic disorders.

Physical Exam

Once your health history has been obtained, the next step is usually a
physical exam. During the physical exam, your height, weight, and
blood pressure will be measured, and other parts of your body will be
checked:

- Ears, eyes, nose, and throat
- Breasts, heart, lungs, and abdomen
- Extremities
- Lymph nodes
- Thyroid
- Skin and teeth

Your reproductive
organs—cervix,
vagina, ovaries,
fallopian tubes,
and uterus—
are checked
during a pelvic
exam. The
initial pelvic
exam is often

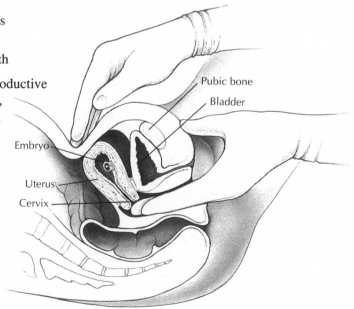

*Your reproductive organs are
felt during a pelvic exam.*

The size of your uterus corresponds to the length of gestation early in pregnancy. It fits inside the pelvis until the 12th week; by the 36th week, the top of the uterus is under your rib cage.

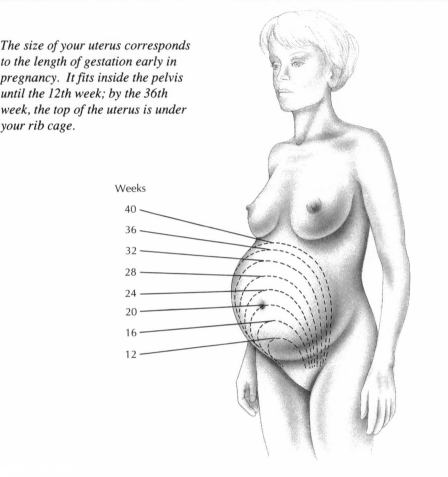

Weeks

40
36
32
28
24
20
16
12

more comprehensive than one done at any other time. Although it can be slightly uncomfortable, this exam is important because the doctor will be checking for changes in your cervix (opening of the uterus) and the size of the uterus.

Early in pregnancy, the size of the uterus corresponds to the length of gestation—the length of pregnancy—and is used as a guide to establishing your due date. Until 12 weeks of gestation, your entire uterus fits inside your pelvis. At midpregnancy (20 weeks of gestation), its top generally reaches the navel. At term, the uterus will be under your rib cage.

When Is the Baby Due?

The average length of pregnancy is 280 days, or 40 weeks, from the first day of the last menstrual period. However, a normal full-term pregnancy can last anywhere between 37–42 weeks of gestation. Only about 5% of babies arrive on the exact due date, and most women deliver within 2 weeks before or after this date.

Estimated Date of Delivery

Based on the information obtained at your first visit, your doctor will calculate your due date, also called the estimated date of delivery, or EDD (also known as the estimated date of confinement, or EDC). The method used most often is based on conception occurring 14 days after the start of the last menstrual period. The approximate date may be figured out by taking the date your last period began, adding 7 days, and then counting back 3 months. For example, if the first day of your last period was May 5, add 7 days to get May 12, then count back 3 months—the estimated due date is February 12. Because it can be difficult to predict the exact date, your doctor may use more than one method:

- If the date of ovulation is known, it is the most reliable method of determining the age of the fetus.
- Throughout pregnancy, but especially early on, a clinical exam, which shows the size of the uterus, can provide useful information.
- Pregnant women usually first feel fetal movements, or *quickening,* by 16–20 weeks.
- In a normal pregnancy, fetal heart tones can usually be heard by the doctor using a special stethoscope by 18–20 weeks, or at 12 weeks by using a *Doppler* device, a form of *ultrasound* that converts sound waves into signals you can hear.
- In the first half of pregnancy, ultrasound can be used to estimate the age of a fetus within 7–10 days. Later in pregnancy, this method is not as accurate.

Calculating the due date on the basis of your menstrual period is not always exact. Menstrual cycles differ from one woman to another, and the pattern of menstrual cycles affects the due date. Also, women often have lapses of memory about their periods. You can help by recording your periods and sharing this information with your doctor.

The Importance of Accuracy

The accuracy of the due date is confirmed by checking the size of the uterus and the regularity, length, and character of the menstrual cycle, including changes in bleeding. If there is doubt about the EDD, ultrasound can be used to confirm or define the date. The due date is important because certain tests, such as ***amniocentesis*** or ***alpha-fetoprotein*** testing (described in "Genetic Tests," Chapter 6), must be done at a specific time in pregnancy and interpreted according to the length of pregnancy in order to get accurate results. The due date is also used as a guide for gauging the growth of the fetus and the progress of your pregnancy—important if the doctor needs to induce labor. If your condition and that of the baby don't correspond with the due date, your doctor can be in a better position to take steps to detect and manage problems if he or she is assured of the accuracy of the due date.

Estimated Date of Delivery

While the average pregnancy is 280 days from the last menstrual period, it is normal to give birth anywhere from 37–42 weeks after your last period. Use this chart to determine your EDD. Locate the **bold-faced** number that represents the first day of your last menstrual period. The light-faced number below it represents the expected delivery date.

Jan	**1**	**2**	**3**	**4**	**5**	**6**	**7**	**8**	**9**	**10**	**11**	**12**	**13**	**14**	**15**
Oct	8	9	10	11	12	13	14	15	16	17	18	19	20	21	22
Feb	**1**	**2**	**3**	**4**	**5**	**6**	**7**	**8**	**9**	**10**	**11**	**12**	**13**	**14**	**15**
Nov	8	9	10	11	12	13	14	15	16	17	18	19	20	21	22
Mar	**1**	**2**	**3**	**4**	**5**	**6**	**7**	**8**	**9**	**10**	**11**	**12**	**13**	**14**	**15**
Dec	6	7	8	9	10	11	12	13	14	15	16	17	18	19	20
Apr	**1**	**2**	**3**	**4**	**5**	**6**	**7**	**8**	**9**	**10**	**11**	**12**	**13**	**14**	**15**
Jan	6	7	8	9	10	11	12	13	14	15	16	17	18	19	20
May	**1**	**2**	**3**	**4**	**5**	**6**	**7**	**8**	**9**	**10**	**11**	**12**	**13**	**14**	**15**
Feb	5	6	7	8	9	10	11	12	13	14	15	16	17	18	19
Jun	**1**	**2**	**3**	**4**	**5**	**6**	**7**	**8**	**9**	**10**	**11**	**12**	**13**	**14**	**15**
Mar	8	9	10	11	12	13	14	15	16	17	18	19	20	21	22
Jul	**1**	**2**	**3**	**4**	**5**	**6**	**7**	**8**	**9**	**10**	**11**	**12**	**13**	**14**	**15**
Apr	7	8	9	10	11	12	13	14	15	16	17	18	19	20	21
Aug	**1**	**2**	**3**	**4**	**5**	**6**	**7**	**8**	**9**	**10**	**11**	**12**	**13**	**14**	**15**
May	8	9	10	11	12	13	14	15	16	17	18	19	20	21	22
Sep	**1**	**2**	**3**	**4**	**5**	**6**	**7**	**8**	**9**	**10**	**11**	**12**	**13**	**14**	**15**
Jun	8	9	10	11	12	13	14	15	16	17	18	19	20	21	22
Oct	**1**	**2**	**3**	**4**	**5**	**6**	**7**	**8**	**9**	**10**	**11**	**12**	**13**	**14**	**15**
Jul	8	9	10	11	12	13	14	15	16	17	18	19	20	21	22
Nov	**1**	**2**	**3**	**4**	**5**	**6**	**7**	**8**	**9**	**10**	**11**	**12**	**13**	**14**	**15**
Aug	8	9	10	11	12	13	14	15	16	17	18	19	20	21	22
Dec	**1**	**2**	**3**	**4**	**5**	**6**	**7**	**8**	**9**	**10**	**11**	**12**	**13**	**14**	**15**
Sep	7	8	9	10	11	12	13	14	15	16	17	18	19	20	21

Routine Tests

Several laboratory tests will be done early in your prenatal care, and some will be repeated at different times during pregnancy:

- *Blood tests* to identify your blood type, Rh factor, and other anti-bodies; to check for anemia and sexually transmitted diseases; and to determine whether you have had German measles (rubella) or have been exposed to hepatitis

	18	19	20	21	22	23	24	25	26	27	28	29	30	31	
7	18	19	20	21	22	23	24	25	26	27	28	29	30	31	**Jan**
4	25	26	27	28	29	30	31	1	2	3	4	5	6	7	Nov
7	18	19	20	21	22	23	24	25	26	27	28				**Feb**
4	25	26	27	28	29	30	1	2	3	4	5				Dec
7	18	19	20	21	22	23	24	25	26	27	28	29	30	31	**Mar**
2	23	24	25	26	27	28	29	30	31	1	2	3	4	5	Jan
7	18	19	20	21	22	23	24	25	26	27	28	29	30		**Apr**
2	23	24	25	26	27	28	29	30	31	1	2	3	4		Feb
7	18	19	20	21	22	23	24	25	26	27	28	29	30	31	**May**
1	22	23	24	25	26	27	28	1	2	3	4	5	6	7	Mar
7	18	19	20	21	22	23	24	25	26	27	28	29	30		**Jun**
4	25	26	27	28	29	30	31	1	2	3	4	5	6		Apr
7	18	19	20	21	22	23	24	25	26	27	28	29	30	31	**Jul**
3	24	25	26	27	28	29	30	1	2	3	4	5	6	7	May
7	18	19	20	21	22	23	24	25	26	27	28	29	30	31	**Aug**
4	25	26	27	28	29	30	31	1	2	3	4	5	6	7	Jun
7	18	19	20	21	22	23	24	25	26	27	28	29	30		**Sep**
4	25	26	27	28	29	30	31	1	2	3	4	5	6	7	Jul
7	18	19	20	21	22	23	24	25	26	27	28	29	30	31	**Oct**
4	25	26	27	28	29	30	31	1	2	3	4	5	6	7	Aug
7	18	19	20	21	22	23	24	25	26	27	28	29	30		**Nov**
4	25	26	27	28	29	30	31	1	2	3	4	5	6	7	Sep
7	18	19	20	21	22	23	24	25	26	27	28	29	30	31	**Dec**
3	24	25	26	27	28	29	30	1	2	3	4	5	6	7	Oct

- *Urine tests* to provide information about levels of sugar and protein and to detect possible infections
- *Pap test* to check for cervical cancer

In addition to routine tests, other tests may also be suggested, depending on your history, family background, or race. Routine screening for diabetes is recommended for women over 29 years old because they are more likely to have the disease, as are women with hypertension, obesity, and other risk factors, regardless of age. Some doctors prefer to screen all women because it is hard to assign an exact age when the risk becomes significant.

The information obtained at your prenatal visits may lead your doctor to suggest further tests to check on the status of the fetus. Some genetic tests may be offered routinely, such as a test to screen for alpha-fetoprotein that detects **neural tube defects** such as **spina bifida**. Others may be recommended, particularly if you have a greater-than-average chance of giving birth to an infant with a birth defect. These tests are discussed in "Genetic Tests," Chapter 6.

Future Visits

After your first prenatal visit, the following visits are usually shorter. The time during these visits is generally used to find out how you are doing and how the baby is growing and to address any special concerns you may have. You and your doctor will work out the timing of these visits, depending on your risk factors. You may follow a schedule somewhat like this one:

From the first visit to 28 weeks. . . . . Monthly
From 28–36 weeks. . . . . Every 2 weeks
From 36 weeks to delivery (at about 40 weeks). . . .Weekly

Women with medical or obstetric problems require more attention, whereas women who have no apparent risk factors may need less. Your doctor will want to see you more often if you have a problem or the potential for developing one.

During these visits, your weight and blood pressure are checked, and a urine sample is taken for testing. Your abdomen is measured to check the growth and position of the fetus, and the fetal heartbeat is checked on each visit. Lab tests and pelvic exams may not be done each time but may be spaced throughout the rest of your visits. These findings, as well as the results of the initial history, physical exam, and tests, will be noted on your medical record.

Throughout your pregnancy, your doctor will give you advice and counseling on leading a healthy life style. You are encouraged to ask questions during your prenatal visits. You should also make a note of any unusual signs or symptoms that may appear between visits. The diary at the back of this book can be used as a handy way to chart the course of your pregnancy (see Appendix A).

Your Medical Record

At your first prenatal visit, your doctor will start keeping a record of your pregnancy and your prenatal care on a form similar to the one in Appendix B. Here is a key to some of the abbreviations you will find there:

AIDS: Acquired immune deficiency syndrome

BCP: Birth control pills

BP: Blood pressure

BR: Breech

CVS: Chorionic villus sampling

DIL: Dilation

EDD: Estimated date of delivery

EFF: Effacement

FHT: Fetal heart tones

FHR: Fetal heart rate

GA: Gestational age

GC: Gonococcal (gonorrhea)

GTT: Glucose tolerance test

HB S Ag: Hepatitis B surface antigen

HCG: Human chorionic gonadotropin

HCT: Hematocrit

HEENT: Head, eyes, ears, nose, and throat

HGB: Hemoglobin

HIV: Human immune deficiency virus

HPV: Human papillomavirus

LMP: Last menstrual period

MCV: Mean corpuscular volume

MSAFP: Maternal serum alpha-fetoprotein

RH : Rhesus blood factor

RhIG: Rhesus immunoglobulin

RX: Treatment, prescription

STA: Station

STD: Sexually transmitted disease

TB: Tuberculosis

UTI: Urinary tract infection

VBAC: Vaginal birth after cesarean

VDRL: Venereal Disease Research Laboratory (syphilis test)

VTX: Vertex

Special Tests

Depending on your history and the results of your routine tests, your doctor may recommend that you have more tests to check the growth and health of the fetus. Some tests, such as ultrasound, allow you and your doctor to see an image of the fetus while it is in your uterus. This can be especially helpful for determining whether your fetus has grown and developed as expected for its age. Other types of tests result in a sound or recording of the fetus's heartbeat. Techniques may be used in combination to create both a sound and an image to assess the well-being of the fetus.

These tests cannot cure a problem, but they can alert your doctor that you may require special care. Although these tests are not fail-proof and so cannot guarantee a healthy baby, they can offer reassurance and help detect potential problems.

Ultrasound

Ultrasound, which creates pictures of the baby from sound waves, is available today in almost every major hospital and in many doctors' offices. This new technology has become useful for the general health care of women, but it is especially valuable during pregnancy and childbirth.

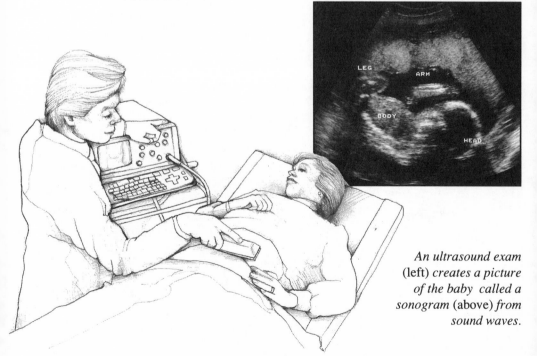

An ultrasound exam (left) *creates a picture of the baby called a sonogram* (above) *from sound waves.*

Ultrasound is energy in the form of sound waves produced by a small crystal. The sound waves move at a frequency too high to be heard by the human ear. They are directed into a specific area of the body through a device called a ***transducer***. The transducer is moved across the skin surface, scanning the area. The sound waves bounce off tissues inside the body, like echoes. They are converted into sounds of the heartbeat of the fetus, or images of the internal organs and the fetus, that appear on a television-like screen. Real-time ultrasound, the type that is used most often, quickly combines still pictures one after another to show movement, somewhat like the individual frames that make a motion picture.

The doctor will decide with you whether to use ultrasound and how often it should be done to best suit your needs. Ultrasound is often used to aid the doctor in detecting a suspected problem or checking a condition that has been confirmed. It can provide information that other tests and procedures do not.

In a way, ultrasound serves as a limited physical examination of a fetus. It can provide valuable information about the fetus's health and well-being, such as:

- Age of the fetus
- Rate of growth of the fetus
- Placement of the ***placenta***
- Fetal position, movement, breathing, and heart rate
- Amount of ***amniotic fluid*** in the uterus
- Number of fetuses
- Some birth defects

To prepare for an ultrasound exam, wear clothes that allow you to expose your abdomen easily, such as a top and a skirt or slacks. Some hospitals may ask you to wear a hospital gown.

A full bladder may be needed for your exam. You may be asked to drink several glasses of water 1 hour before the exam and not to urinate until after the procedure. A full bladder serves as a landmark, helping the doctor locate the pelvic organs. It also allows clearer, more accurate pictures. With ultrasound, the only discomfort you feel is that of a full bladder.

A doctor or an ultrasound technologist, someone specially trained in performing ultrasound exams, will conduct the test. As you lie on the table with your abdomen exposed from the lower part of the ribs to the hips, mineral oil or a gel is applied to the surface of the abdomen to improve contact of the transducer with the skin surface. The transducer is then moved along the abdomen. The sound waves sent out from the transducer enter the body and are reflected back when they come into contact with the internal organs and the fetus. The transducer may also be inserted in the vagina to aid in viewing the pelvic organs.

Although the effects of ultrasound are still being studied, no harmful effects to either the mother or the baby have been found in over 20 years of use. The long-term risks of ultrasound, if any, are unknown, but there are many benefits.

Fetal Heart Rate Monitoring

Ultrasound can be used to listen to the fetus's heartbeat. Sound waves are transmitted via an instrument that is held against the mother's abdomen or attached there with belts. Monitoring the fetus's heart can help show how it is responding to labor (see "Monitoring," Chapter 13) and also can give some helpful information before labor.

There are two types of electronic fetal monitoring that your doctor may use during pregnancy to check on the fetus. The *nonstress test* measures the fetus's heart rate in response to its own movements. The *contraction stress test* measures the fetus's response to contractions.

Nonstress Test. Usually the fetal heart rate increases when the fetus moves. The nonstress test measures the response of the fetus's heart rate to each of its movements, as felt by the mother or noted by a doctor or nurse. The heart rate is noted on a paper recording. If the fetus does not move for a short time during the test (perhaps as long as 40 minutes), it may be because it is asleep. If this happens, your doctor may try waking the fetus by using a buzzer.

The nonstress test may be combined with ultrasound to give a *biophysical profile*. The biophysical profile is most often used for women who are at increased risk of having a complicated pregnancy because of a medical condition such as high blood pressure or diabetes. The biophysical profile examines the fetus's breathing movements, muscle tone, body movement, and the amount of amniotic fluid (the liquid surrounding the fetus inside the uterus). Each of these items is given a score, and the total is added. As with electronic fetal monitoring, the biophysical profile does not cause any harm to the fetus, so it can be repeated weekly, if necessary, to check on the progress of your pregnancy. Your doctor may use the score to decide whether you need special care or whether your baby should be delivered early.

Electronic fetal monitoring can be used to check the heart rate of the fetus.

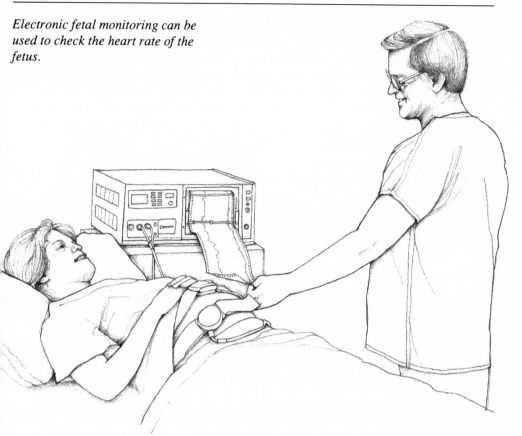

Contraction Stress Test. The contraction stress test measures how the fetal heart rate reacts to the temporary decrease in blood flow to the placenta that occurs during a uterine contraction. A normal response to this test implies that the fetus is receiving enough oxygen at the moment. This does not necessarily predict whether the fetus will respond well to future stress or labor, however. An abnormal response indicates the need for further testing and possibly treatment.

This test is often used if the nonstress test shows no change in fetal heart rate in response to fetal movement. Mild contractions of the mother's uterus are brought on by giving a drug called *oxytocin* or having the mother stimulate her nipples. The fetus's heart rate in response to the contractions is then recorded.

Risk Factors

A pregnancy is considered to be at increased risk when a problem is more likely than usual to occur. Such a problem could be caused by a health condition that the mother had before she was pregnant, or it may arise during pregnancy or at delivery. The small number of women who have recognized risks account for a large number of the problems that occur. Not all complications of pregnancy can be predicted, however. About 20% of infants who are in poor health or who die are born to mothers who did not have any signs of risk during pregnancy.

Factors That Can Complicate Your Pregnancy

Medical

- Hypertension
- Heart, kidney, lung, or liver diseases
- Infections—sexually transmitted diseases, urinary tract infections, or other viral or bacterial infections
- Diabetes
- Severe anemia
- Convulsive diseases, such as epilepsy

Obstetric

- Problems in past pregnancies
- Mother younger than 15 or older than 35 years old
- Previous birth defects
- Multiple gestation (eg, twins or triplets)
- Bleeding, especially during the second or third *trimester*
- Pregnancy-induced high blood pressure (*preeclampsia*)
- Abnormal fetal heartbeat
- Intrauterine growth retardation or prematurity (fetus not developed adequately for age)

Life Style

- Smoking
- Drinking alcohol
- Taking drugs not prescribed by physician (either illegal or over-the-counter drugs)
- Poor nutrition, including inadequate weight gain
- Lack of prenatal care
- Multiple sexual partners

Because problems can arise at any time, risks will be assessed throughout the pregnancy. Regardless of when problems occur, they can threaten the health of the mother or that of the fetus, or both. For this reason, a woman with an increased risk of complications will require more intensive prenatal care.

Questions to Consider...

- Is there anything in my history I may have overlooked that could pose a problem in pregnancy?
- When is my due date?
- What are the dates of my future visits?
- Will I need any special tests?

Chapter 6

Genetics

Genetics is the study of how traits are passed on from parents to a child. Many personal traits are inherited this way, such as height and eye color. Unfortunately, some diseases can be passed on in the same way. A condition that affects a fetus and is present at birth is called a *congenital disorder*. Through counseling and testing, you may be able to learn whether your fetus is at risk for having certain genetic diseases and congenital disorders.

Genes and Chromosomes

Egg ⊗   Sperm ♂

The fetus inherits 23 chromosomes each from its mother and father to make 23 pairs. The twenty-third pair determines the sex of the fetus: XX is female and XY is male.

Male ♂

Normally, each male sperm and each female egg contain 23 gene-carrying chromosomes, or one-half of the 46 found in all other cells in the body. When an egg is fertilized by a sperm, the 23 chromosomes from the mother's egg and the father's sperm join to form the 46 chromosomes of the fetus. One pair of the chromosomes—one each from the sperm and the egg—are the sex chromosomes. There are two types of sex chromosomes, designated by the letters X and Y. A normal sperm will carry either an X or a Y; a normal egg is always X. If the union of an egg and a sperm is an XY, the child will be male; if XX, female. A man's sex chromosome thus decides the sex of his child.

Each chromosome carries many genes. Genes are responsible for the traits a person inherits from his or her parents. Genes come in pairs. Each parent contributes one-half of each pair of chromosomes and, thus, half the genes. Although some traits are controlled by a single gene pair, others, including eye and hair color, are the result of many pairs of genes working together.

Genetic Disorders

Although most children in the United States are born healthy, about 2–3% of babies are born with some type of major congenital birth defect. Another 4–5% of babies are born with less serious problems, some barely noticeable or easily corrected. Although the cause of a birth defect is not always known, the cause of many genetic disorders is now well understood.

Dominant Gene Disorders

A dominant disorder needs only one gene from either parent to cause an effect on the child. The chances are 50–50 that any child (male or female) of this parent will inherit the gene. Following are some of the disorders that are passed on by a dominant gene:

- *Polydactyly* (having extra fingers or toes) is fairly common and can be corrected by surgery.
- *Achondroplasia* is a very rare abnormality of the skeleton in which a person has shorter-than-normal arms and legs. Most often it is the result of a new mutation, meaning that neither parent has the trait. When both parents are affected and each passes on the abnormal gene, the disorder is fatal.
- *Huntington disease* (a problem with the nervous system that causes uncontrollable movements and mental deterioration) usually affects people in their 30s or 40s. Each child of a person with Huntington disease has a 50% chance of having the disorder.

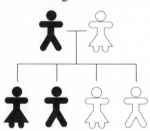

If one parent has a dominant gene disorder, there is a 50% chance that it will be passed to each child.

Recessive Gene Disorders

A genetic disorder can occur when a pair of the fetus's genes is made up of two abnormal recessive genes—one from each parent. Because there are so many genes within each cell, everyone carries a few abnormal recessive genes. Yet, in most people, no defect appears because the abnormal recessive gene is overruled by the normal gene.

In certain groups, it is more likely that the parents will both carry the same abnormal gene. For example, recessive disorders are more

If both parents are carriers of a recessive disorder, there is a 25% chance that a male or female child will be affected and a 50% chance that a child (boy or girl) will be a carrier and not have the disorder.

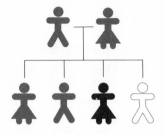

common in certain ethnic groups and in relationships between blood relatives. It is for this reason that marriages between first cousins and other near relatives are discouraged.

If both parents have a recessive disorder, all their children will have the disorder, too. If one parent has the disorder and the other does not (and isn't a carrier of the abnormal gene), all their children will be carriers, but none will have the disorder. Following are some common recessive disorders:

• *Cystic fibrosis* is the most common genetic disease among white persons of northern European descent. It causes the respiratory system to produce very thick mucus, clogging the lungs and causing lung disease. Most individuals with cystic fibrosis are infertile. Cystic fibrosis most often affects infants, children, and young adults. In the United States, the chance of a white person having the disease is about 1/2,500, and the chance of being a carrier is 1/25. For black Americans, the risk is only 1/17,000 for the disease and 1/50 for being a carrier. By testing a person suspected of having the cystic fibrosis gene and his or her relatives, it is possible to identify carriers of the gene and most fetuses who have the disease.

• *Sickle cell disease* affects mostly black persons. In the United States, about 1 in 625 blacks are affected, and about 1 in 10 are carriers. With sickle cell disease, the red blood cells take on a crescent, or "sickle" shape, rather than the normal "doughnut" shape. The abnormal, sickle-shaped red blood cells tend to get caught in the blood vessels, cutting off oxygen to tissues and causing pain. Because the body destroys these abnormal cells faster than it can make normal ones to replace them, anemia often occurs. Both carrier tests of the parents and prenatal tests of the fetus are available.

• *Tay–Sachs disease* is found mostly in persons whose families are of eastern European Jewish descent (Ashkenazi Jews). In this group, the disease occurs in 1 in 3,600 births. The chance of being a carrier is 1/30 for Ashkenazi Jews, but 1/300 for other persons. Symptoms first occur at about 6 months of age, progressively causing severe mental retardation, blindness, seizures, and death within a few years. Both tests for carriers and prenatal tests of the fetus are available.

- *Beta-thalassemia* causes anemia and is more likely to occur in persons of Mediterranean descent, such as Italians and Greeks. The risk for beta-thalassemia in these populations is between 1/2,500 and 1/800. The chance of being a carrier is about 1/25. Both carrier testing and prenatal testing of the fetus are available.

X-Linked Disorders

Some genetic disorders are determined by genes on the X chromosome and are thus referred to as X-linked or sex-linked. In most of these disorders, the abnormal gene is recessive. A woman can carry such a gene on one of her X chromosomes, yet not have the disorder because her normal gene on the other X chromosome prevents the disorder from being expressed. Because a male child will get one of his mother's X chromosomes, he may be affected. If the mother is a carrier for one of these X-linked disorders and the father is normal, there is a 50% chance that any given son will have the disorder and a 50% chance that any of their daughters will be a carrier. Very rarely, a daughter can inherit certain X-linked recessive disorders if, for example, her father and mother both have the disease.

Hemophilia is an X-linked disease. Persons with hemophilia lack a substance needed for blood clotting. Internal bleeding can be life-threatening to people with hemophilia, because they are very slow to stop bleeding. Hemophilia occurs in about 1 in 2,500 male babies. Testing a sample of blood will show whether an individual has hemophilia, and prenatal testing of the fetus is available.

Chromosomal Disorders

Genetic disorders may also be caused by problems with the fetus's chromosomes. Some of these are inherited, but most are caused by an error in the development of the egg or sperm. Having extra or missing chromosomes, or parts of chromosomes, usually causes serious

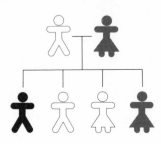

If a woman is a carrier of an X-linked (or sex-linked) disorder, there is a 50% chance that she will pass the disorder to her son and a 50% chance that her daughter will be a carrier.

medical problems. Most children born with chromosome disorders are mentally retarded in addition to having physical defects. The risk of having a child with a chromosomal abnormality increases with the age of the mother. The chance that a 35-year-old woman will have a child with any type of chromosomal abnormality is about 1 in 200; for a 40-year-old woman, the chance is about 1 in 60. Chorionic villus sampling or amniocentesis (described later) can identify fetuses with chromosomal disorders before birth.

Of the disorders affecting one of the autosomal chromosomes, Down syndrome is the most common. Like other chromosomal disorders, the risk increases with the age of the mother: it is 1 in 1,667 live births for 20-year-old mothers, 1 in 378 live births for 35-year-olds, and 1 in 106 live births for 40-year-olds. Affected children are

Risk of Having a Baby with Chromosomal Disorders

	Risk of Having a Live Baby with:	
Mother's Age	Down Syndrome	Any Chromosomal Disease
20	1/1,667	1/526
21	1/1,667	1/526
22	1/1,429	1/500
23	1/1,429	1/500
24	1/1,250	1/476
25	1/1,250	1/476
26	1/1,176	1/476
27	1/1,111	1/455
28	1/1,053	1/435
29	1/1,000	1/417
30	1/952	1/385
31	1/909	1/385
32	1/769	1/322
33	1/602	1/286
34	1/485	1/238
35	1/378	1/192
36	1/289	1/156
37	1/224	1/127
38	1/173	1/102
39	1/136	1/83
40	1/106	1/66
41	1/82	1/53
42	1/63	1/42
43	1/49	1/33
44	1/38	1/26
45	1/30	1/21
46	1/23	1/16
47	1/18	1/13
48	1/14	1/10
49	1/11	1/8

mentally retarded and have a characteristic facial appearance. Persons with Down syndrome usually have three (called trisomy) number 21 chromosomes instead of the normal two. Trisomy can also occur with other chromosomes: numbers 13 and 18, for example. These children are severely retarded and have many physical defects.

Other chromosomal disorders can occur when a person has too many or too few sex chromosomes. Men can have either an extra X chromosome or an extra Y chromosome. Males with Klinefelter syndrome have an extra X chromosome—that is, two X chromosomes and one Y chromosome. They have testicles that are smaller than normal and may be infertile; some are mentally retarded. Klinefelter syndrome affects about 1 in 800 men. Slightly less common is having one X chromosome and two Y chromosomes. Men with an extra Y chromosome may be taller than normal.

Women can have just one X chromosome (Turner syndrome). Women with Turner syndrome tend to have puffiness of the hands and feet and webbing at the back of their necks. They may have incomplete development of their secondary sex characteristics, but early hormone treatment can help modify this. They are almost always infertile. The risk for Turner syndrome is about 1/3,000.

Multifactorial Disorders

Many disorders are thought to be somehow the result of multifactorial inheritance—a mix of genetic and environmental factors. The frequency of these disorders may vary in different parts of the world. Some can be detected in pregnancy, but most cannot. A couple who has a child with a disorder of multifactorial inheritance usually has a 1–5% chance of having the disease affect future children. Two common multifactorial disorders are congenital heart defects and neural tube defects.

Congenital heart defects occur in about 1 in 125 infants. Although there are other causes of congenital heart defects, such as infection with rubella virus (German measles) or a specific chromosome problem, about 90% of the time these defects are the result of multifactorial inheritance. Congenital heart defects can sometimes be identified before birth by *ultrasound*. In most cases, if parents have one child a with congenital heart defect, their chance of having another child with a heart defect is about 2–4%.

Neural tube defects occur when the tube enclosing the spinal cord does not close completely or form properly. In the very early stages of pregnancy, a long, narrow groove forms on the surface of the embryo, eventually deepening and then closing around itself to form a tubelike structure. It is from this neural tube that the spinal cord will develop, with the brain forming at one end. Only 1–2 pregnancies per 1,000 result in babies born with a neural tube defect.

The two major types of neural tube defects are ***anencephaly*** and ***spina bifida***. Anencephaly occurs when the brain and head do not develop normally. Because the upper part of the brain is absent or underdeveloped, babies with this disorder are almost always ***stillborn*** or die shortly after birth.

Spina bifida has been called "open spine," because sometimes when the lower part of the neural tube doesn't close during embryo development, the spinal cord and nerve bundles are exposed outside the baby's body. This defect can be fatal, or it can result in serious long-term problems.

The other form of spina bifida, in which the defect is covered with skin, can also result in handicaps. However, they occur less often and are usually less severe than those associated with open spina bifida. With surgery and physical therapy, many children with a mild neural tube defect can lead relatively normal and productive lives.

The following disorders also can be passed on through multifactorial inheritance:

- *Clubfoot*—The affected foot is twisted at the ankle.
- *Cleft lip and palate*—A gap or space in the lip or a hole in the palate (roof of the mouth). When parents have already had a child with a cleft lip and palate, they have about a 4% chance of having another affected child. If they have had a child with cleft palate alone, they have a 2% chance of having another affected child.
- *Hip dislocations*—The ball and socket of the hip joint do not fit together well. This occurs more often in girls than in boys.

Counseling

Certain couples have a higher risk of having a baby with a birth defect. These include couples who have already had a child with a birth defect or who have a history of genetic disorders in their family. Women aged 35 and older are also at risk, as are couples of certain ethnic and racial backgrounds. If you are at increased risk of having a genetic disorder, genetic counseling is recommended. As a part of the counseling, you will be asked to recall family medical histories as far back as possible. This will help your doctor or a geneticist (someone who has special training in genetics) to determine your risk for various diseases. Certain tests also can show whether your fetus is affected.

The results of exams, tests, and histories will be explained, and the risk of a birth defect will be calculated. No test is 100% accurate, however. Your fetus may have a birth defect even if the test for it is negative or may be free of that defect even if the test is positive.

Less than 3% of all babies are born with a birth defect. Some defects are more likely to recur if you have already had one child with that defect.

The information you learn through genetic testing and counseling can help you make some important choices. If you or your partner is found to be a carrier of a genetic disorder, you will want to know what the risk is that the disorder may be passed on to any child you decide to have. Depending on the circumstances, you may choose to build your family by adoption. If the father is a carrier of a genetic disorder and the mother is not, you may want to consider artificial insemination, which is described in Chapter 2.

Risk of Genetic Disorders

Disorder	Risk of Having a Fetus with the Disorder	
	Overall	With One Affected Child
Dominant gene		
Polydactyly	1/300–1/100[1]	50%
Achondroplasia	1/23,000	50%
Huntington disease	1/15,000–1/5,000	50%
Recessive gene		
Cystic fibrosis	1/2,500[2]	25%
Sickle cell anemia	1/625[1]	25%
Tay–Sachs disease	1/3,600[3]	25%
Beta-thalassemia	1/2,500–1/800[4]	25%
X-linked		
Hemophilia	1/2,500 men	50% for boy, 0% for girl
Chromosomal		
Down syndrome	1/800[5]	1–2%
Klinefelter syndrome	1/800 men	N/S[6]
Turner syndrome	1/3,000 women	N/S[6]
Multifactorial		
Congenital heart disease	1/125	2–4%
Neural tube defects	1–2/1,000	2–5%
Cleft lip/cleft palate	1/1,000–1/500	2–4%

[1]Black persons.
[2]White persons.
[3]Ashkenazi Jews.
[4]Persons of Mediterranean descent.
[5]Average risk increases with mother's age.
[6]No significant increase.

Genetic Tests

Based on your personal medical history, your family medical history, and other factors, your doctor may offer certain special procedures or tests to detect genetic disorders. These tests are not cures, nor can they be expected to detect all potential problems. A specific test can be used to identify a specific problem, however, giving valuable information about the risk to your fetus.

In addition to the procedures described, there is a new method called percutaneous umbilical cord blood sampling (PUBS), in which a sample of the fetus's blood is checked for some diseases. This technique has risks, is very new, and may not be available in your area.

Alpha-Fetoprotein

Some tests are used to screen pregnant women for a disorder regardless of whether they have any risk factors. Measuring a chemical called *alpha-fetoprotein (AFP)* by a simple blood test can help identify women who might be carrying a fetus with a neural tube defect, a condition that often arises without warning. This test is called maternal serum AFP (or MSAFP) screening.

AFP is a protein produced by every growing fetus. Some of this protein is passed into the *amniotic fluid* that surrounds the developing fetus inside the mother's uterus. A smaller amount crosses the *placenta* (or afterbirth) into the mother's blood. When the fetus has an open neural tube defect, large amounts of AFP leak into the amniotic fluid and then into the mother's blood. When the defect is covered by skin, however, the AFP is less likely to leak into the amniotic fluid. This type of neural tube defect is harder to detect by AFP testing or ultrasound. Low AFP levels have also been linked to a possible increased risk of Down syndrome.

For the MSAFP test, a small amount of blood is taken from the mother's arm. It is recommended that MSAFP testing be performed between 15–18 weeks of pregnancy. In order to interpret the MSAFP test properly, it is important to establish the age of the fetus as accurately as possible. Timing is also important for another reason: if the first test results are positive (higher or lower than would be expected at that point in pregnancy), enough time must remain in the pregnancy for further steps in the testing process.

If the results of the first blood test are negative, no further tests are needed. Yet this is no guarantee. Neural tube defects or Down syndrome may occur with negative test results. The AFP test can be a useful indicator. It will identify 90% of fetuses with anencephaly (lacking a brain) and 75% of those with spina bifida (having an opening in the back that exposes the spinal cord). It will identify about 25% of fetuses with Down syndrome in women under age 35.

For every 1,000 women tested, about 50 have an elevated AFP test. Of these 50, only 1–2 with higher-than-normal tests are carrying fetuses with a neural tube defect. Other possible causes for a positive test include incorrect dating of pregnancy, twins, or other conditions relating to high levels of AFP. Positive first test results, for whatever reason, mean that further testing is necessary. Those women whose test results are positive are offered further counseling and testing, which may include ultrasound and amniocentesis.

Amniocentesis

In *amniocentesis,* a sample of amniotic fluid is withdrawn through a needle. The amniotic fluid is then tested for certain genetic disorders. Amniocentesis is usually done at 14–18 weeks of pregnancy and can be performed on an outpatient basis, either in a hospital or in the doctor's office.

For the procedure, the patient is asked to lie down on an examining table, and her abdomen is uncovered. With the aid of ultrasound, a slender needle is carefully guided through the abdomen into the uterus and the amniotic sac. A small sample (about 1 ounce) of fluid is withdrawn through the needle (this fluid is replaced in a short time). This fluid is sent to a laboratory for testing. A number of fetal cells will be present in the amniotic fluid. The fetal cells in the fluid are grown in a special culture and then analyzed. The specific tests that are done will depend on your personal and family medical history.

During amniocentesis, a small sample of amniotic fluid is withdrawn to be studied.

Amniotic fluid is also tested for the level of alpha-fetoprotein as another means of detecting birth defects.

It can take about 2–4 weeks for enough fetal cells to grow so that a diagnosis can be made. These cells are prepared in such a way that their chromosomes can be studied under a microscope. The presence of an extra chromosome (as occurs in Down syndrome) or other chromosomal abnormalities can be diagnosed by such study. Because the sex of the fetus is also revealed by the test, amniocentesis may be used to help determine the risks of a sex-linked disorder.

Although complications from amniocentesis are uncommon, there is some risk involved. Occasional side effects include cramping, vaginal bleeding, and leaking of amniotic fluid after the procedure. Injury to the fetus is rare.

Miscarriage (loss of a pregnancy before the fetus is able to survive outside the uterus) occurs in about 3% of all pregnancies from 16 weeks of pregnancy onward, even if amniocentesis is not performed. With amniocentesis, the risk of miscarriage is increased up to about 0.5%.

Chorionic Villus Sampling

Chorionic villi (singular, villus) are microscopic, finger-like projections that make up the placenta. Villi come from the same fertilized

Amniotic Fluid

The fetus develops inside a sac formed by two membranes, the amnion and the chorion. Inside the sac, a liquid called amniotic fluid collects to support and protect the fetus. This watery environment in which the fetus grows is always changing: new amniotic fluid is being formed constantly, and some of the old is swallowed by the fetus.

Amniotic fluid begins forming during 4–5 weeks of pregnancy. At first it is composed almost entirely of fluid from the mother. As early as 11 weeks, the fetus's kidneys start to produce a weak urine. From midpregnancy onward, the fetus's urine is the main source of the fluid.

Amniotic fluid cushions the fetus, distributing evenly any shocks to the mother's abdomen. Because the fluid exerts pressure on the walls of the uterus, the fetus has room to grow. In a safe, temperature-controlled environment, the fetus can practice the movements it will need after birth. It can exercise its muscles by moving around, and as it breathes in and swallows the fluid it develops both a swallowing and a breathing mechanism. Amniotic fluid also discourages the growth of some kinds of bacteria, helping to protect the fetus from infection.

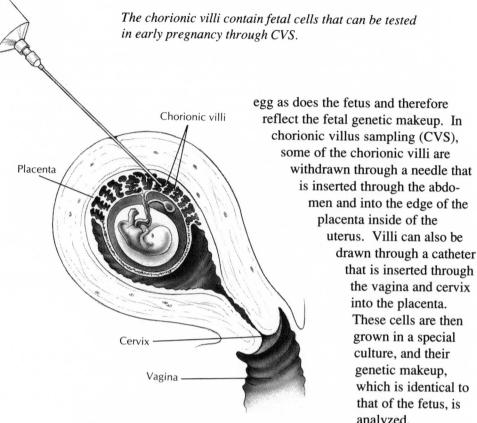

The chorionic villi contain fetal cells that can be tested in early pregnancy through CVS.

Chorionic villi

Placenta

Cervix

Vagina

egg as does the fetus and therefore reflect the fetal genetic makeup. In chorionic villus sampling (CVS), some of the chorionic villi are withdrawn through a needle that is inserted through the abdomen and into the edge of the placenta inside of the uterus. Villi can also be drawn through a catheter that is inserted through the vagina and cervix into the placenta. These cells are then grown in a special culture, and their genetic makeup, which is identical to that of the fetus, is analyzed.

In contrast to amniocentesis, which is performed in the second *trimester* of pregnancy, CVS can be performed during the first trimester, allowing for earlier detection of genetic defects. The results can be obtained more quickly—within about 10 days—allowing a diagnosis to be made, usually before the end of the first trimester.

As with amniocentesis, there are some risks with CVS. The most common complication is miscarriage. The risk of this happening is still fairly low, though—up to 1% higher than if CVS isn't done.

Abnormal Test Results

If one or more of your genetic tests has been positive, then the chance of your having a baby with a defect is increased. The facts and your feelings should be discussed with your partner, doctors, and counselors. This is often a difficult time for couples expecting a baby. Counseling can be very helpful in determining why your fetus is at risk for this disease and what options you have now and in the future.

If you are carrying a fetus with a genetic defect, you are faced with a difficult choice: You can choose either to end the pregnancy or to begin preparing for the birth of the child. This decision requires a great deal of thought, and often it may have to be made more quickly than you would like. Every couple has a different set of resources and values, so a decision that is right for one couple may not be right for another.

If you decide that the best course for you is to end the pregnancy in an abortion, it will most likely be done soon. The earlier the abortion is done, the simpler and safer it is for the woman.

Other couples elect to continue the pregnancy and have the baby. If you decide to have the baby, it is helpful to use the time remaining in the pregnancy to prepare yourself and your family. You may want to read about the condition your child may have or to join a support group. Along with your doctor and your family, you may start to plan the best possible care for your child beginning at birth. It may be difficult to predict how severely affected the child will be. Regardless of the decision you make, you may find counseling helpful in coming to terms with these issues.

Questions to Consider...

- What is the chance of my baby having a genetic disorder?
- Could my partner or I be a carrier of a genetic disorder?
- Should I have an alpha-fetoprotein test or amniocentesis?
- Should I have amniocentesis or CVS?

Chapter 7

A Healthy Life Style

Many of the choices you make in your daily life affect your fetus. This is true of the things you do—exercise, rest, and work—as well as the things you don't do—expose your fetus to drugs, alcohol, cigarettes, or other risks. Some women may need to change their life style during pregnancy. This change may not be easy, but your doctor and the health care team can give you information and support. Even better is the daily support of your family and friends, and especially your partner. Together, you can construct a healthy life style that will benefit you and your baby.

Exercise

Regular exercise during pregnancy can lead to a better appearance and posture, enhance your feeling of well-being, and lessen some of the discomforts of pregnancy, such as backache and tiredness. The goal of exercise during pregnancy should be to reach or keep a level of fitness that is safe.

What you can do in sports and exercise during pregnancy depends on your own health and, in part, on how active you were before you became pregnant. This is not a good time to take up a new, strenuous sport, but if you were active before your pregnancy, you should be able to continue, within reason. Caution should be the rule.

Here are some general guidelines for following a safe and healthy exercise program geared to the special needs of pregnancy:

- Regular exercise (at least three times per week) is better than spurts of heavy exercise followed by long periods of no activity.
- Brisk exercise should not be performed in hot, humid weather or when you have an illness with a fever, such as a cold or flu.
- Avoid jerky, bouncy, or high-impact motions. Activities that require jumping, jarring motions, or rapid changes in direction may cause pain. Exercise on a wooden floor or a tightly carpeted surface to reduce shock and provide a sure footing. Wear a good-fitting, supportive bra to help protect your breasts.
- Avoid deep knee bends, full sit-ups, double leg raises, and straight-leg toe touches. During pregnancy, these exercises may injure the tissue that connect your leg and back joints.

Prenatal Exercises

There are a number of exercise programs designed especially for pregnant women. You doctor can help you select exercises that are best for you.

Head and Shoulder Circles

Slowly moving your head and shoulders in circles can help relieve upper backache and tension in your head, neck, and shoulders.

- Stand or sit in a comfortable position.
- Inhale while slowly dropping your head toward your left shoulder and circling it to the back and on toward your right shoulder.
- Exhale while slowly letting your head circle to the front and around to your left shoulder again.
- Repeat several times.

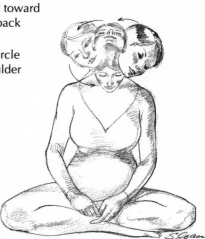

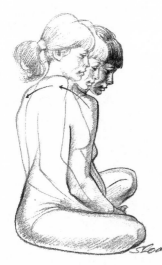

- Inhale while slowly moving your right shoulder forward and then upward to form the top half of a circle.
- Exhale while slowly moving your shoulder to the back and then down to complete the circle.
- Repeat with your left shoulder.
- Do three to five repetitions.

Forward Bend

This exercise stretches and relaxes the muscles in your back to help relieve tension and fatigue.

- Stand with your feet about 12–18 inches apart and your knees slightly bent. (As you do this exercise, spread your legs, bend your knees, or do both, as needed for comfort. Don't try to keep your knees straight.)
- Exhale and bend forward from the waist, letting your upper body slowly sag toward the floor, uncurling slowly.
- Inhale and slowly uncurl your back, one vertebra at a time, until you are once again standing up straight. (Do not try to keep your back straight or to rise quickly to a standing position, because you may become dizzy.)

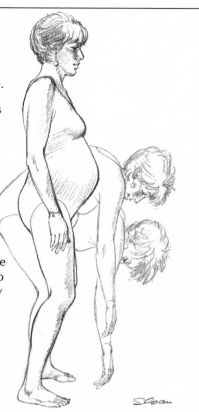

Arm Reaches

Stretching your side and upper body helps relieve upper backache. It is also helpful when you feel short of breath.

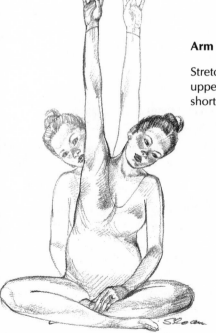

- Stand or sit in a comfortable position.
- Inhale as you raise your right arm above your head, reaching as high as you can. (Be sure to stretch from the waist, without letting your hip or foot rise.)
- Exhale, bending your elbow and pulling your arm back down to your side.
- Repeat on your left side.
- Do three to five repetitions.

Pelvic Tilt

Tilting your pelvis back towards your spine can help strengthen your abdominal muscles and relieve backache. This exercise can be done in either a kneeling or standing position.

Standing

- Stand in a comfortable position.
  - Inhale and relax.
    - Exhale as you roll your hips and buttocks forward, as if trying to lift the fetus up toward your chest.
  - Hold for a count of five.
  - Inhale and relax.
  Repeat three to five times, several times a day.

Kneeling

- Kneel on your hands and knees, with your back relaxed but not arched.
- Inhale and relax a moment.
- Exhale and pull your buttocks under and forward (you should feel your abdomen tighten and your back straighten at the waist).
- Hold for a count of five.
- Inhale and relax.

Side Leg Stretches

This exercise improves your circulation and tones and strengthens the muscles of your hips, buttocks, and thighs.

- Lie on your left side, with your knees, hips, and shoulders in a straight li Put your right hand on the floor in front of you, and use your left hand t support your head.
- Inhale and relax.
- Exhale while slowly raising your right leg as high as you can without bending your knee or body. Keep your foot flexed, with your right outs ankle bone facing up.
- Inhale while slowly lowering your leg.
- Repeat 10 times.
- Turn to your right side and repeat 10 times with your left leg.

Leg Stretches

Stretching your legs relieves tension in your hips and legs and helps relieve or prevent leg cramps.

- Sit on the floor with your right leg stretched out toward the side, your foot flexed, and your left leg folded in.
- Facing forward, lean your upper body to the right side, so that your right ear is directly over your right leg. At the same time, lift your left hand over your head, so that it is directly over your left ear.
- Using your right hand, grasp your right foot—or your ankle or calf if you cannot reach your foot comfortably.
- Hold this position for a count of 10.
- Relax and release the stretch.
- Repeat on the left side.
- Do three times (as you feel more comfortable with this exercise, try to hold the stretch longer).

You can change this exercise two different ways for more variety:

1. Instead of raising your leg all the way up, raise it only halfway and make small circles with it. Make 10 clockwise circles and then 10 counterclockwise circles.

2. Instead of keeping your upper leg straight, bend your knee so that your upper thigh is at a right angle to your body. Keeping your knee bent, do the side raises, making sure that your knee faces forward and your outer ankle bone faces upward.

- Avoid exercises that require lying with your back on the floor for more than a few minutes after 20 weeks of pregnancy.

- Always begin with a 5-minute period of slow walking or stationary cycling with low resistance to warm up your muscles. Intense exercise should not last longer than 15 minutes.

- Heavy exercise should be followed by a 5–10-minute period of gradually slower activity that ends with gentle stretching in place. To reduce the risk of injuring the tissue connecting your joints, do not stretch as far as you possibly can.

- The extra weight you are carrying will make you work harder as you exercise at a slower pace. Measure your heart rate at peak times of activity (see "Exercise," Chapter 1). Do not exceed your target heart rate and limits established with your doctor's advice.

- Get up slowly and gradually from the floor to avoid dizziness or fainting. Once you are standing, walk in place for a brief period.

- Drink water often before and after exercise to prevent dehydration (lack of enough water for the body's needs). Take a break in your workout to drink more water if needed.

- Women who did not regularly exercise before becoming pregnant should begin with physical activity of very low intensity and move to higher levels of activity very gradually.

- Stop your activity and consult your doctor if any unusual symptoms appear, such as the following:

  —Pain
  —Bleeding
  —Dizziness
  —Shortness of breath
  —Palpitations (irregular heartbeat)
  —Faintness
  —*Tachycardia* (rapid heartbeat)
  —Back pain
  —Pubic pain
  —Difficulty walking

Almost any form of exercise is safe if it is done in moderation. Some exercises offer aerobic conditioning of the heart and lungs; others relieve stress and tone muscles. Pregnancy causes many changes in your body, some of which have an effect on your ability to exercise. These changes can interfere with activities that require good balance, so you may wish to modify your form of exercise during pregnancy.

- *Walking* is always good exercise. If you were not active before you became pregnant, walking is a good way to begin an exercise program.

- *Swimming* can be continued if you were used to swimming before pregnancy. Swimming is excellent for your body because it uses many different muscles while the water supports your weight. However, it is best not to dive in the later months of pregnancy. Scuba diving is not recommended during pregnancy.

- *Jogging* can be done in moderation if you were used to jogging before you became pregnant. Avoid becoming overheated, stop if you are feeling uncomfortable or unusually tired, and drink water to replace what you lose through sweating.

- *Tennis* is generally safe if you were used to playing tennis before pregnancy, but be aware of your change in balance and how it affects rapid movements.

- *Golf and bowling* are fine for recreation but don't really strengthen the heart and lungs. With either of these sports, you may have to adjust to your change of balance.

- *Snow skiing, water skiing, and surfing* pose some risk. You can hit the ground or water with great force, and taking a fall at such fast speeds could harm you or your fetus. Before you decide to participate, you should talk with your doctor.

Sex

Most couples can continue to have intercourse until shortly before the baby is born. Sometimes couples are afraid that the act of intercourse will harm the fetus and cause a *miscarriage*—this is not true. The fetus is well cushioned by the *amniotic fluid* surrounding it.

For your comfort, you and your partner may want to try different sexual positions. For example, intercourse with the man and woman on their sides causes less pressure on the woman's abdomen and limits how far the man's penis can extend into the vagina.

Although the basic guide to intercourse during pregnancy is your own comfort, there are a few reasons your doctor may advise you to limit or avoid having intercourse:

- Past miscarriage or *preterm* birth
- Infection
- Bleeding
- Pain
- Breaking of the amniotic sac or leaking amniotic fluid

Intercourse is not the only form of sexual expression. Other forms of expressing your sexuality can be equally satisfying. This is an area that you may wish to discuss with your doctor.

Whatever form of sexual expression you choose, it's best to stay with one steady partner. A monogamous relationship, in which both partners are faithful to each other, is more important now than ever. Women who have more than one sexual partner greatly increase their chances of getting a sexually transmitted disease. These diseases are dangerous for the mother and the fetus (see "Sexually Transmitted Diseases," Chapter 1).

Harmful Agents

Teratogens are agents that can cause birth defects when a woman is exposed to them during pregnancy. Hazards can be posed by drugs that are prescribed, chemicals that occur in the environment or work place, or infections (see Chapter 12). These agents can interfere with the normal development of the fetus, resulting in physical and mental defects (other agents are suspect, but have not been proven to be harmful). Their effect depends on the fetus's stage of development when exposure occurred and the dosage received. Other substances, such as tobacco and illicit drugs, are harmful in different ways and should be avoided for the sake of your health and that of your baby.

Work-Related Hazards

The risk of exposure to many of the substances that occur in the work place is not known. Scientific information is either lacking or conflicting. A few of the substances that can be found in the work place, however, are known to cause harm.

Heavy metals, such as lead and mercury, are teratogens. Lead is used in some industries. Tollbooth attendants and others who work on heavily traveled roads may also be exposed to high levels of lead.

Ionizing radiation is used to take X-rays of the internal organs to diagnose a problem. It can also be used in larger doses for treatment. In larger doses, such as those used to treat cancer, it can harm a fetus. Most women who work around radiation, however, are protected against exposure.

CAUTION RADIOACTIVE MATERIAL

The radiation from color television sets, video display terminals (VDTs), and microwave ovens is known as nonionizing radiation. Persons working near these sources are not exposed to dangerous levels of radiation. In the last 10 years, however, it has been suggested that the radiation from VDTs causes problems during pregnancy. VDTs, also called cathode-ray tubes (or CRTs), create both ionizing radiation, which is absorbed by the glass screen, and nonionizing radiation, which can escape from the back of the unit. More studies are needed to determine for certain whether this affects the fetuses of pregnant VDT users.

If you think that you may be exposed to a hazardous agent through your work, talk to your employer about it. You may be able to be moved to another job on a temporary basis.

Medications

Any type of medicine can affect the fetus, and some can cause severe birth defects or other problems for the baby. Don't stop taking any medication prescribed by a doctor—the lack of treatment could be more harmful than the drug—but do seek medical advice.

Be sure that the doctor caring for you during pregnancy knows about any medical problems you may have. Tell him or her about any drugs other doctors have prescribed for you and whether you have any drug allergies. You may need to change the kind or amount of drug you take.

Not all drugs require a prescription. Products such as pain medicines (aspirin, acetaminophen, or ibuprofen), cold and allergy medicine, and some skin treatments are drugs, even though you can buy them in a drug store without a prescription. Over-the-counter

Agents That Can Harm the Fetus

Agent	Reasons Used	Effects
Alcohol	Part of regular diet, social reasons, dependency	Growth and mental retardation
Androgens	To treat endometriosis	Genital abnormalities
Anticoagulants, eg, warfarin (Coumadin, Panwarfin) and dicumarol	To prevent blood clotting; used to prevent or treat thromboembolisms (clots blocking blood vessels)	Abnormalities in bones, cartilage, and eyes; central nervous system defects
Antithyroid drugs, eg, propylthiouracil, iodide, and methimazole (Tapazole)	To treat an overactive thyroid gland	Underactive or enlarged thyroid
Anticonvulsants, eg, phenytoin (Dilantin), trimeth-adione (Tridione), paramethadione (Paradione), valproic acid (Depakene)	To treat epilepsy and irregular heartbeat	Growth and mental retardation, developmental abnormalities, neural tube defects
Chemotherapeutic drugs, eg, methotrexate (Mexate) and aminopterin	To treat cancer and psoriasis (skin disease)	Increased rate of miscarriage, various abnormalities
Diethylstilbestrol (DES)	To treat problems with menstruation, symptoms of menopause and breast cancer, and to stop milk production; previously used to prevent preterm labor and miscarriage	Abnormalities of cervix and uterus in females, possible infertility in males and females
Lead	Industries involving lead smelting, paint manufacture and use, printing, ceramics, glass manufacturing, and pottery glazing	Increased rate of miscarriage and stillbirths
Lithium	To treat the manic part of manic–depressive disorders	Congenital heart disease
Organic mercury	Exposure through eating contaminated food	Brain disorders

Agents That Can Harm the Fetus *(continued)*

Agent	Reasons Used	Effects
Isotretinoin (Accutane)	Treatment for cystic acne	Increased rate of miscarriage, developmental abnormalities
Streptomycin	An antibiotic used to treat tuberculosis	Hearing loss
Tetracycline	An antibiotic used to treat a wide variety of infections	Underdevelopment of tooth enamel, incorporation of tetracycline into bone
Thalidomide	Previously used as a sedative and a sleep aid	Growth deficiencies, other abnormalities
X-ray therapy	Medical treatment of disorders such as cancer	Growth and mental retardation

drugs should not be taken during pregnancy without checking first with your doctor. Instructions that come with these over-the-counter drugs are usually not meant for a pregnant woman.

Illicit Drugs

The life style that often goes with the use of illicit drugs often makes it difficult to pinpoint their effects during pregnancy. It is known, however, that drug users are more likely to have problems during pregnancy that place their babies at risk. The effects of drugs can be so harmful that even occasional users are at risk.

Marijuana is the illicit drug that is used most often. Women who are moderate or heavy users (two to five uses per week) tend to deliver early, and their babies are often small. Marijuana can be retained in the body for long periods, leading to prolonged fetal exposure, and it contains carbon monoxide, a gas that could keep the fetus from receiving enough oxygen.

Cocaine, the second most often used illicit drug, is especially dangerous during pregnancy. It can be snorted, injected, or smoked in a highly purified and addictive form known as crack. Cocaine abuse is more harmful than any other substance abuse in pregnancy. Pregnant women who use cocaine have a 25% higher chance of having a preterm birth. Their babies are at risk for being small for their age and are often more irritable and fussy. Cocaine can cause the mother to have a heart attack and could cause death of the fetus. Recent studies suggest that even babies who survive being exposed to cocaine during pregnancy will have long-lasting physical, behavioral, and emotional problems.

Other illicit drugs, such as heroin, methadone, and phencyclidine (PCP or angel dust), can be addictive to the baby as well as the mother. When these babies are born, they must go through withdrawal from the drug.

Addictions can be hard to quit. Pregnancy may give you extra incentive to try. If you want to stop using illegal drugs, talk to your doctor. He or she can give you more information about the effects of these drugs on your fetus and can refer you to a treatment program.

You should try to stop taking any drugs as soon as possible. The fetus's organs form during the first *trimester*, and using drugs during this time can cause serious damage to these organs. Cutting down on or stopping drug use anytime in pregnancy, however, does provide some benefits.

Smoking   When a pregnant woman smokes, she risks not only her own health but that of her baby. Smoking hurts the baby before, during, and after birth. Each puff exposes the fetus to harmful chemicals. Carbon monoxide travels to the fetus's blood. This lowers the amount of oxygen to both the mother and the fetus. Nicotine crosses the *placenta* (which connects mother and fetus) and can cause the fetal blood vessels to constrict so that less oxygen and nourishment reach the fetus.

Smoking increases a woman's risk of complications during pregnancy. Pregnant smokers are more apt to have vaginal bleeding during pregnancy. They are also more likely to have a miscarriage, *stillbirth*, or preterm baby (born before 37 weeks). On the average, a smoker's baby weighs ½ pound less than a nonsmoker's baby and is about ½ inch shorter in body length. Low birth weight raises the baby's chances of being born early and needing special care. *Sudden infant death syndrome (SIDS)* occurs more than twice as often among babies of smoking mothers.

The sooner you quit, the better it will be for your baby. If you stop smoking during the early months of your pregnancy, your chance of having a low-birth-weight baby will be close to that of a non-smoker. Almost one-fourth of all pregnant women quit smoking while they are pregnant. If you cannot stop smoking, you can still help your fetus by smoking as little as possible. If you can quit during pregnancy, you can quit for a lifetime, and it will be a healthier one.

Alcohol   About 60% of American women drink alcoholic beverages. There is a difference between alcohol *use* and alcohol *abuse*. Some people have one or two drinks on various occasions—this is alcohol use. Others may drink daily or in binges (drinking a large amount of alcohol in a short time)—this is alcohol abuse. The amount of alcohol that separates use from abuse is not clearly defined.

When a pregnant woman drinks alcohol, it quickly reaches the fetus through the bloodstream. The same level of alcohol that goes through the mother's bloodstream also goes through the fetus's. A number of studies have been done on infants born to women who drank heavily during pregnancy. Many of the infants were born with a strong pattern of physical, mental, and behavioral problems. This group of problems is called fetal alcohol syndrome.

Babies that had the syndrome were shorter and lighter in weight than normal babies and did not catch up, even after special care was provided. They also had small heads; abnormal features of the face, head, joints, and limbs; heart defects; and poor control of movement. Most were mentally retarded and showed a number of behavioral problems, including hyperactivity, extreme nervousness, and poor attention span. Some of the infants were born with all of these problems; others showed signs of only some of them.

Other factors—cigarette smoking, use of other drugs, poor diet, problems handling stress—may well play a role in fetal alcohol syndrome. But alcohol itself appears to be the one common agent in all cases. Other factors alone cannot account for the damage.

It appears that the more a mother drinks during pregnancy, the greater the danger to the fetus. The fetus is especially at risk early in pregnancy, when all of the major body systems are being developed. Alcohol increases the risk of having a miscarriage at this time. The risk is about twice as high in pregnancies complicated by maternal drinking, although perhaps only among women who drink heavily.

One of the questions asked most often about alcohol and pregnancy is whether there is a safe level of alcohol intake. Does the woman who drinks only once in a while put her baby in danger? There is no evidence that an occasional drink is harmful. Women who have an occasional drink seem to have babies with no more problems than those women who drink rarely or not at all.

Moderation is the key. Avoid binges and daily drinking. That type of drinking is more dangerous. Even if you don't binge and you believe your drinking is moderate, it's still best to try to cut down. Reducing intake anytime during pregnancy can be beneficial.

It is hard to state how much alcohol puts the fetus at risk. Each fetus may be affected differently. It is best to cut down gradually over

Do You Have a Drinking Problem?

Sometimes it can be hard to tell the difference between alcohol use and alcohol abuse. Experts in treating alcohol abuse use the CAGE questions to help them find out whether a person has a drinking problem:

C Have you ever felt you ought to **cut down** on your drinking?
A Have people **annoyed** you by criticizing your drinking?
G Have you ever felt bad or **guilty** about your drinking?
E Have you ever had a drink first thing in the morning to steady your nerves or to get rid of a hangover? Ever had an **eye-opener**?

If you answer "yes" to any of these questions, or if you notice an increased tolerance to drinking, you may have a problem with alcohol. Talk to your doctor about your drinking habits. He or she can give you more information and refer you for counseling or treatment.

a 6-month period before you become pregnant. Because it isn't known how much alcohol is harmful, the safest course is to drink alcohol rarely or not at all during pregnancy. It's just one more way to change your life style in order to increase your chances of having a healthy, normal baby.

The Battered Woman

Abuse of women by their male partners—physical, sexual, or emotional abuse—is one of America's most widespread health problems. It can occur regardless of socioeconomic or ethnic group, race, age, or religion. The consequences of this abuse are serious. About 20% of the visits made by women to emergency rooms are for injuries related to abuse. Over one-third of female murder victims are killed by their male partners. Children may also be affected, because men who abuse their partners often also abuse their children.

Abuse often begins or increases during pregnancy, putting both the mother and the fetus at risk. During pregnancy, the abuser is more likely to direct his blows at the woman's breasts and abdomen. Dangers to the fetus include miscarriage, low birth weight, and direct injury from blows to the mother's abdomen. Sometimes, though, abuse decreases during pregnancy. In fact, some women feel safe only when they are carrying a child. This can lead to repeated pregnancies as a way of escaping abuse.

There are better ways of dealing with abuse, though. First, realize that you are not to blame for your partner's actions. Abusers blame their victims, but it is not your fault. He and he alone is the cause of his actions. Second, tell someone you trust about your situation—a close friend, doctor or nurse, counselor, or a clergy member. Letting someone else know can be a relief, and the person you tell can help you get in touch with support services such as crisis hot lines, domestic violence programs, legal aid services, or shelters for battered women and children. Counseling can help you to understand the situation and to make a decision about what to do.

The next step is ensuring your safety and the safety of any children you have. Make a rapid-action plan that will allow you and your children to leave quickly, if needed. Some steps you may want to follow include:

- Pack a suitcase to store with a friend or neighbor. Include a change of clothes for you and your children and an extra set of keys to the house and car.

- Keep important items in a safe place so you can take them with you on short notice—prescription medicines; identification such as birth certificates, social security cards, and driver's license; cash, a checkbook, savings account book, and credit cards; and a special toy for each child.

• Know exactly where you will go and how to get there at any time of the day.

• Know what you will do if you can't escape the violence—go to the doctor or emergency room, tell the doctor how you were hurt, and ask for a copy of your medical record in case you want to file charges later.

• Call the police—physical abuse is a crime, even if you are living with or married to the abuser.

Learn to recognize the signs of impending danger so you can use your exit plan to avoid a violent incident. These can include your male partner having a weapon or threatening to use one, threatening or hurting children or other members of the family, forcing you to have sex, or showing less guilt and remorse after he is violent.

No one deserves to be abused: not you, not your fetus, and not your children. If your male partner has begun or continues to abuse you, talk to someone and start taking steps to end the violence.

Work

Today more than 51 million women make up almost half of America's work force. Of these, more than 1 million become pregnant each year. Many of these women work until a short time before delivery and return to work within weeks or months of the baby's birth. This trend, along with a growing awareness of on-the-job health and safety, has prompted women, doctors, and employers to ask a number of questions that have no easy answers: Is it safe for a pregnant woman to work? How long, under what conditions, and with what effects can she continue to work?

If your job is strenuous or requires a lot of standing or walking, your doctor may ask you to cut back on work hours, transfer to less strenuous work, or stop working a few weeks before delivery. Your doctor may also advise you to stop working if you have certain diseases, have given birth to more than one premature baby, have a history of miscarriages, or are expecting more than one baby. Otherwise, if you are a normal, healthy woman—with an uncomplicated pregnancy and a normally developing fetus—and you work in a job that presents no greater hazards than those in daily life, you can usually work until your due date.

Pregnancy-Related Disability

Having a disability means that you are not able to work because of physical problems that could interfere with your ability to perform your usual duties. Only you and your doctor can decide whether your pregnancy is partially or totally disabling. A disability may fall into any of three categories:

1. *Disability of the pregnancy itself.* Some women suffer side effects such as nausea, vomiting, indigestion problems, dizziness, and swollen legs and ankles during pregnancy. Your doctor should reevaluate these minor problems at regular intervals.

2. *Disability related to complications.* More serious complications, such as infection, bleeding, or early rupture of the amniotic sac, may cause disability. Also, medical conditions you had before becoming pregnant, such as heart disease, diabetes, or high blood pressure, may be disabling during pregnancy.

3. *Disability related to job exposure.* Some disabilities may be job related, linked with such factors as exposure to high levels of toxic substances.

If your doctor decides that your pregnancy is disabling, you may request a letter to verify to your employer that you are eligible for disability benefits. Likewise, if your doctor says you are able to keep working, your employer may request you (or you may choose) to submit a letter from your doctor stating so.

Disability Benefits for Pregnant Employees

Employee maternity policies vary widely from company to company and state to state. Only about 40% of employed women in the United States are entitled to paid 6-week disability leave for childbirth. Others must use sick leave and vacation time or take time off without pay.

The Pregnancy Discrimination Act, passed by Congress in 1978, requires employers offering medical disability compensation to treat pregnancy-related disabilities in the same manner as all other disabilities. It means that if you are temporarily unable to work because of pregnancy, your employer must give you the same rights as other employees temporarily disabled by illness or accident. If you are partially disabled by pregnancy and your employer regularly assigns lighter work to other partially disabled workers, the same must be done for you. Unfortunately, many employers offer no disability benefits at all and therefore are not obligated to provide maternity leave.

If no disability plan is offered where you work, you may qualify for unemployment or temporary disability benefits from your state. To find out whether your state offers benefits and how to qualify, contact your local unemployment office.

Pregnant women can usually keep doing the physical activities they are used to doing. Heavy lifting, climbing, carrying, and other efforts requiring agility and stamina may cause discomfort for some. These and long hours may pose a risk.

The first few months of pregnancy may bring periods of dizziness, nausea, fatigue, and heat sensitivity that can increase the risk of accidents. Toward the end of pregnancy, you become more vulnerable to falls because your body balance changes with your increase in

Your Rights As an Employee

The 1978 Pregnancy Act is an amendment to the Civil Rights Act of 1964. This act requires your employer to offer the same medical disability compensation for pregnancy-related disabilities as is offered for other disabilities.

The Occupational Safety and Health Administration (OSHA) in Washington, DC (phone: 202-634-7460), administered under the Department of Labor, was created under the Occupational Safety and Health Act of 1970. OSHA sets and enforces standards requiring employers to provide a work place free from recognized hazards causing, or likely to cause, death or serious physical harm and to provide information to employees about dangerous chemicals and substances. State and municipal statutes also give employees and unions the right to request the names of chemicals and other substances used in the work place. At the request of an employee, union, or health care provider, OSHA representatives will perform work place inspections.

The National Institute for Occupational Safety and Health (NIOSH) in Atlanta (phone: 404-331-2396) operates under the Department of Health and Human Services. While OSHA is in charge of regulation in the work place, NIOSH is responsible for research—identifying hazards, figuring out ways to control them, and recommending federal standards to limit the dangers. At the request of an employee, union, or health care provider, NIOSH investigates health and safety standards in the work place.

weight and abdomen size. Also, because women tire more easily when pregnant, even those in the best physical condition will find strenuous labor more tiring than usual.

At home, housework and child care duties don't stop during pregnancy and can also be strenuous work. More responsibilities may need to be shared at this time with your partner or others to ensure you are getting enough rest.

Travel

Travel during pregnancy is generally safe if you make certain allowances and preparations. The most comfortable time in pregnancy for most women to travel is during the second trimester (14–28 weeks of gestation). By this time, your body has adjusted to pregnancy, and you

The Right Way to Wear a Safety Belt

For the best protection, you should wear a lap–shoulder belt throughout your pregnancy every time you travel in a car, including during your ride to the hospital for the birth of your baby. Some cars have only lap belts in the back seat. If a lap belt is all that is available, use it.

Place the lower part of the lap–shoulder belt under your abdomen, as low as possible, and against your upper thighs. Never place the belt above your abdomen, because this could cause major injuries in a crash. Position the upper part of the belt between your breasts. Adjust both the upper and lower parts of the lap–shoulder belt as snugly as possible.

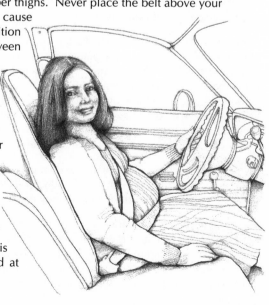

The belt should cross your shoulder without chafing your neck. Never slip the upper part of the belt off your shoulder. Safety belts worn too loosely or too high on the abdomen can cause broken ribs or injuries to your abdomen. But more damage is caused when they aren't used at all.

probably have more energy. Morning sickness is usually no longer a problem during these months, and the rate of complications is at its lowest.

The best method of transportation when you are pregnant is very often the one you enjoy most. There are some hints that apply no matter what type of transportation you choose:

- You will be more comfortable if you stop frequently and walk around. Try to walk around and stretch every hour and a half.
- Be sure to wear comfortable clothing that doesn't bind.
- Take some crackers or other light snacks with you to help prevent nausea.
- Traveling can upset your stomach and disrupt your sleeping habits and your health. Do not take any medications—either prescription

---

Foreign Travel: Let the Traveler Beware

If you are thinking about taking a trip out of the country, discuss your plans with your doctor. He or she can help you decide whether foreign travel would be safe for you, and if so, what steps you should take in advance.

Traveling to other countries exposes you to diseases that are not common in the United States. Natives of a country are used to the organisms found in the food and water, but the same organisms can make a visitor ill. This is true whether you travel to cities or rural areas.

Although traveler's diarrhea may be a minor nuisance to a nonpregnant traveler, it is a greater concern for a pregnant women. The best way to avoid getting diarrhea is by avoiding contaminated food and water. Iodine used to purify water may not be safe for pregnant women. Drink only pure bottled water, bottled soft drinks, hot tea, or broth. Don't use ice in your drinks, and avoid using glasses that could have been washed in contaminated water. Instead, drink out of the bottle or use paper cups. Avoid fresh fruits and vegetables unless they have been cooked or can be peeled.

If you do get diarrhea, drink plenty of pure water and other fluids. Do not take any medicine without checking with a doctor first. There are some medicines safe for treating diarrhea during pregnancy that a doctor can prescribe.

Malaria is a tropical infection passed on by mosquito bites. It produces flu-like symptoms and anemia. Complications of malaria are more common in pregnant women, and malaria increases the risk of miscarriage, stillbirth, and small babies. Avoiding mosquito bites by wearing long-sleeved clothing and using mosquito netting, bug repellant, or lotion is the best way to avoid malaria.

drugs or over-the-counter preparations—without checking with your doctor. This includes anti-motion-sickness pills and laxatives.

- Take a copy of your prenatal record with you.
- Ask your doctor to recommend another doctor who can care for you at your new location if you plan to be away from home for an extended time.
- Check with your doctor about the chance of premature labor if you plan to travel very late in pregnancy.

Although travel during pregnancy is considered safe in most cases, it is not recommended for women who have serious health problems that need special medical care. If you are unsure about whether travel is safe for you, ask your doctor.

Although no drug completely protects you against malaria, chloroquine is effective in preventing and treating most cases. It is safe for use in pregnancy. You must start taking it before you travel and continue afterwards for a few weeks. You should not plan to travel to areas where there are mosquitoes that carry strains of malaria that are resistant to chloroquine (such as East Africa and Thailand), because there is no other safe drug that prevents malaria.

Immunization is often not required by law for travel, but depending on where you plan to go, it may be a good idea. Ideally, vaccines should be given before you become pregnant, but some can be given during pregnancy. As a rule, though, live vaccines should not be given during pregnancy (see Chapter 12). You and your doctor will need to decide whether the risks of a disease are greater than the risks of its vaccine. In some cases it may be best to postpone a trip until after pregnancy.

By Land

Traveling by car can be a good choice, especially if you're traveling a short-to-medium distance. If you travel by car, be sure to wear your seat belt. Some women worry that the belt will squeeze the fetus if the car stops quickly or if there is an impact, but this is very unlikely. Inside the uterus, which is protected by muscles, organs, and bones, the fetus is cushioned in a fluid-filled sac. Studies have shown that in nearly 100% of car crashes, the fetus recovers quickly from any pressure the seat belt exerts and suffers no lasting injury. The risk of *not* wearing a seat belt includes being thrown from the car or receiving a concussion, an injury to the brain that is caused by a hard blow. These risks are much more serious than any from wearing a seat belt.

Buses may not allow much room to move around, and stops will be farther apart than if you were driving. When traveling long distances, trains may allow you more freedom of movement than buses.

By Air

Flying is generally safe during pregnancy. Airlines in the United States usually allow pregnant women to fly up to 36 weeks of pregnancy. Commercial airplanes are pressurized, but many private planes are not. It is best to avoid altitudes greater than 7,000–9,000 feet in unpressurized airplanes.

When flying, try to get an aisle seat (in the forward part of the cabin for a more stable ride) so you can get up and move around and have easy access to the bathroom. You should try to stand and walk in the aisle or do leg lifts. Eat lightly to avoid airsickness. Special meals are available on many flights if you order in advance. The metal detectors used for airport security checks are not harmful to the fetus.

By Sea

Boat cruises can be a slow, often relaxing way to travel. Still, travel by boat may present special concerns. If you are thinking about taking a cruise, you might want to discuss some of these issues with your doctor:

• Medicine you can take for seasickness
• Distance from medical care while the cruise is on the open sea
• Special diet concerns

Questions to Consider...

- Can I continue my present exercise program?
- Do my partner and I need to change our sexual practices during pregnancy?
- What can I do to remove myself and my fetus from harmful agents or situations?
- Is it safe for me to work while I'm pregnant? How long should I plan to be off work?
- Should I alter my travel plans while I'm pregnant?

Chapter 8

Nutrition

Eating habits and choices are personal. What you eat is influenced by family, attitudes, beliefs, and taste preferences, as well as by food availability and price. It is hard to adopt a new diet if other family members are not sharing it, if it is disagreeable, or if it means giving up lifelong traditions and habits. It is important that you examine the foods in your daily diet and be alert to their content, how they provide nutrition to your fetus, and how they provide the calories for your own needs and energy. Usually major changes are not necessary to meet the nutritional needs of pregnancy. Women from many cultures, with many different food habits, have healthy babies. The total number of calories and the content of what is eaten are the most important factors.

A Healthy Diet

The Four Food Groups

A way to determine whether you are eating a balanced diet is to use the concept of food groups. Certain types of food are better sources for specific nutrients than others. On the basis of their similarity, some foods can be classified into groups. Selecting portions of food from each of these groups on a daily basis is a reliable way to be sure that you are eating a balanced, wholesome, and healthy diet.

If you use this guide in planning your meals, you will probably be getting enough protein, calories, fats, carbohydrates, and vitamins and minerals in your diet. If you are worried about your diet, keep a record of everything you eat for 24–48 hours. Show your doctor your record, or look up the foods you ate in a book that lists the nutrients in common foods.

Essential Nutrients

Every diet should include proteins, carbohydrates (sugars and starches), fats, vitamins, and minerals. All of these nutrients are complex chemicals that your body uses for growth and repair. The table at right shows how much you need of each of the basic elements before pregnancy, during pregnancy, and when breast-feeding. To be sure that your diet gives you the right amounts of these food elements, you need to know which foods are good sources.

When you look at the labels on boxes, cans, and bottles, you'll often see the initials RDA. This stands for Recommended Daily Allowance. RDAs are nutritional standards created on the basis of available scientific knowledge by a committee of the National Academy of Sciences, a nongovernmental institution. These recommendations are intended to meet the needs of almost every healthy person. If you consume less than the daily RDAs, it does not necessarily mean that you have an inadequate diet. However, if your diet provides nutrients in amounts equal to or greater than the RDAs, it is very likely that you are eating appropriately.

Protein

Proteins are made of long strings of chemicals called amino acids. The body can produce all but 8 of the 22 amino acids that it needs for health and growth. The 8 amino acids the body can't produce are sometimes called the essential amino acids, because they must be provided by what you eat.

Recommended Daily Dietary Allowances for Adolescent and Adult Nonpregnant, Pregnant, and Lactating Women*

Nutrient (unit)	Nonpregnant			Pregnant	Lactating
	15–18 yr	19–24 yr	25–50 yr		
Protein (g)	44	46	50	60	65
Calcium (mg)	1,200	1,200	800	1,200	1,200
Phosphorus (mg)	1,200	1,200	800	1,200	1,200
Magnesium (mg)	300	280	280	320	355
Iron (mg)	15	15	15	30	15
Zinc (mg)	12	12	12	15	19
Vitamin A (µg)	800	800	800	800	1,300
Vitamin D (µg)	10	10	5	10	10
Vitamin E (mg)	8	8	8	10	12
Vitamin C (mg)	60	60	60	70	95
Thiamin (mg)	1.1	1.1	1.1	1.5	1.6
Riboflavin (mg)	1.3	1.3	1.3	1.6	1.8
Niacin (mg)	15	15	15	17	20
Vitamin B_6 (mg)	1.5	1.6	1.6	2.2	2.1
Folic acid (µg)	180	180	180	400	280
Vitamin B_{12} (µg)	2	2	2	2.2	2.6

* Adapted from *Recommended Dietary Allowances,* © 1989, by the National Academy of Sciences National Academy Press, Washington, DC.

Daily Food Needs

Group 1: Fruits and Vegetables

- Fights off infections; promotes healthy skin and good eyesight
- Provides vitamins and minerals
- Four or more daily servings needed
- Select one serving rich in vitamin A (dark yellow or green, leafy vegetables: broccoli, spinach, greens, carrots, winter squash) and one serving rich in vitamin C (citrus fruit, tomatoes, or other fruit, such as cantaloupe or strawberries)

Group 2: Whole-Grain or Enriched Bread and Cereal

- Provides energy and fiber to avoid constipation
- Provides carbohydrates, vitamins, minerals, and protein
- Four or more daily servings needed

Group 3: Milk and Milk Products

- Builds bones and teeth; aids growth of new tissue and repair of body cells
- Provides calcium, phosphorus, protein, and vitamins
- Four or more daily servings needed
- If you don't like milk, substitute items made from milk, such as yogurt, cottage cheese, sliced cheese, or custard

Group 4: Meat, Poultry, Fish, Eggs, Nuts, and Beans

- Helps build new body tissue; prevents anemia
- Provides protein, iron, and vitamins
- Three or more daily servings needed
- Organ meats, such as liver and kidneys, are particularly good. Be sure to add a little cheese, milk, or meat to meals with main dishes made of dry beans, peas, nuts, lentils, or other legumes.

Protein provides nutrients needed to grow, maintain, and repair body tissues such as muscles. It is also needed to make hemoglobin, the chemical that carries oxygen in the blood and gives blood its red color; *antibodies*, which fight infection; and other chemicals the body must produce. Protein should make up no more than 15% of the average adult woman's diet.

Adults and all but the youngest children should eat 45 grams (a little over 11/2 ounces) of high-quality protein each day. High-quality protein comes from animals—meats, fish, poultry, milk, and other dairy products. Examples of animal foods rich in proteins include roast beef, ham, and canned tuna (3-ounce servings each provide 27 grams of protein), broiled chicken (3 ounces provides 22.5 grams of protein), and low-fat milk (1 cup provides 11.25 grams of protein).

Plant products such as grains and legumes can also be good sources of protein. Because they don't contain all the needed amino acids, however, they must be carefully paired with other foods to provide a complete source of protein. Grains or legumes can be paired with animal proteins (cheese pizza, meat chili with beans, or milk and cereal) or with each other (black-eyed peas and rice, peanut butter sandwich, or lima beans and corn) to provide a more complete source of protein.

Vitamins and Minerals

Nutrient	Functions in Body	Food Sources
Vitamins		
A	Needed for normal vision in dim light; prevents eye diseases; needed for growth of bones and teeth	Green, leafy vegetables; dark yellow vegetables (eg, carrots and sweet potatoes); whole milk; liver
Thiamine (B_1)	Helps body digest carbohydrates; needed for normal functioning of nervous system	Whole-grain or enriched breads and cereals; fish, pork, poultry, lean meat; milk
Riboflavin (B_2)	Helps body release energy to cells; promotes healthy skin and eyes	Milk; whole-grain or enriched breads and cereals; liver; green, leafy vegetables
B_6	Helps form red blood cells; helps body use protein, fat, and carbohydrate	Beef liver, pork, ham; whole-grain cereals; bananas
B_{12}	Maintains nervous system; needed to form red blood cells	Liver, meat, fish, poultry; milk (found only in animal foods—vegetarians should take a supplement)

Vitamins and Minerals *(continued)*

Nutrient	Functions in Body	Food Sources
Vitamins *(continued)*		
C	Speeds healing of wounds and bones; increases resistance to infection; needed to form collagen (flexible tissue that helps support body)	Citrus fruits (eg, oranges, lemons, grapefruit); strawberries; broccoli; tomatoes
D	Helps body use calcium and phosphorus; needed for strong bones and teeth	Fortified milk; fish liver oils (you also get vitamin D when you're out in the sunshine)
E	Needed for use of vitamin A; helps body form and use red blood cells and muscles	Vegetable oils; whole-grain cereals; wheat germ; green, leafy vegetables
Folic Acid	Needed to produce blood and protein; helps some enzymes function	Green, leafy vegetables; dark yellow fruits and vegetables; liver; legumes and nuts
Niacin	Promotes healthy skin, nerves, and digestion; helps the body use carbohydrates	Meat, liver, poultry, fish; whole-grain or enriched cereals
Minerals		
Calcium	Needed for strong bones and teeth; helps in blood clotting; needed for normal muscle and nerve function	Milk and milk products; sardines and salmon with bones; collard, kale, mustard, and turnip greens
Iodine	Needed to produce hormones that regulate body's energy use	Seafood; iodized salt
Iron	Needed to make hemoglobin; prevents anemia; increases resistance to infection	Red meat, liver; dried beans and peas; enriched cereals; prune juice
Magnesium	Needed for nerve and muscle function; helps body use carbohydrates	Legumes; whole-grain cereals; milk; meat; green vegetables
Phosphorus	Needed for strong bones and teeth	Milk and milk products; meat, poultry, fish; whole-grain cereals; legumes
Zinc	Needed to produce some enzymes and insulin	Meat; liver; oysters and other seafood; milk; whole-grain cereals

Carbohydrates

Sugars provide the body's main source of energy. There are two types of sugar. The simple sugars, like *glucose*, are ready to be used by the body right away and thus provide the quickest form of energy. Sources of this type of sugar are table sugar, honey, syrup, and hard candies. Often this type of sugar is found in many processed foods.

The other type of sugar is starches. They are the storage form of simple sugars and are a long-lasting energy source. Examples of foods that contain starches are grains, fruits, and vegetables. Other good sources are bread, rice, pasta, and starchy vegetables such as potatoes or corn.

Foods rich in starch also provide fiber, the tough part of plants that gives them support. Although your body cannot digest most kinds of fiber, it is still useful. Fiber speeds your digestion and helps keep you "regular." Fiber can also help your body rid itself more quickly of extra amounts of cholesterol and fats.

Carbohydrates should make up the largest part of a healthy diet, 55% or more of the total. (There is no U.S. RDA for carbohydrates.) Simple sugars do not provide many other nutrients, so they should be just a small part of your diet. Rely more on starches, which provide both energy and fiber. You should eat about 20–30 grams (about 1 ounce) of fiber each day.

Fats

Fats are either saturated or unsaturated. Saturated fats, which are often solid at room temperature, come from animal sources (for example, butter) and some vegetable fats. Palm oil and coconut oil are vegetable fats high in saturated fats. Unsaturated fats tend to be liquid at room temperature (oils) and come mostly from plants and vegetables. Fish oil is also unsaturated.

Fats provide a very concentrated source of energy. This also means they are high in calories. For example, while a gram of protein or carbohydrate provides 4 calories, a gram of fat provides 9 calories. In addition to providing energy, fats also help the body use vitamins A, D, E, and K (the fat-soluble vitamins), proteins, and carbohydrates. Any extra fat not used by the body is stored as fat tissue, to be used later when energy is needed.

Fats should make up no more than 30% of the average diet. Saturated fats should make up no more than one-third of your total fat consumption, or no more than 10% of your total calories.

Obvious sources of fat are the butter, margarine, lard, shortening, and cooking oil that you cook with or put on your food. However, fat is a part of many other foods as well—meats, baked goods, and even nondairy coffee creamer. Choose unsaturated fats more often and saturated fats less often. For example, choose corn oil margarine instead of butter. Remember, though, that even if a package is labeled "no cholesterol" or "contains no animal fat," it could still contain saturated fats such as palm oil.

Although meats can be high in fat, they are one of your best sources of protein. There are ways you can get the protein you need while limiting the fat. Choose lean meats, fish, or poultry and low-fat or skim milk. Trim the fat you can see on meat and remove chicken skin (where most of the fat is found) before cooking. Use low-fat cooking methods such as broiling, baking, or poaching.

Vitamins and Minerals

Vitamins and minerals are essential for the body's health. The best way to get all the vitamins and minerals you need is through a balanced diet. Sometimes, though, there may be special reasons why you can't get all the nutrients you need from your diet. To help you get the vitamins and minerals you need, your doctor may recommend supplements. You should not take more than the U.S. RDA amount of vitamins unless your doctor prescribes them.

Water

Water is not often thought of as a nutrient, but life cannot exist without it. It is used to build new tissue, carry nutrients and waste products, aid digestion, and help chemical reactions. One-half to three-fourths of your body's weight is water. In addition to the water that is used by your body, some is lost through sweat and urine. To be sure that your body is getting enough water, you should drink six to eight glasses of liquids each day. Choose water, fruit juices, and milk more often. Because they contain simple sugars and caffeine, choose coffee, tea, and sodas less often.

Nutritional Needs During Pregnancy

During pregnancy your body has special nutritional needs that must be met. Because you are doing all the fetus's digestion and breathing, you will need more energy and thus must consume more calories. Your body also needs to produce more blood to be able to circulate some through the *placenta*. This means you will need more iron, protein, and folic acid. Growing fetal bones require additional minerals, such as calcium and phosphorus. If you already have a balanced diet, then it is a simple matter to add the extra nutrients that are needed for the fetus.

Calories and Weight Gain

Both your weight before you get pregnant and the amount of weight you gain during pregnancy determine the baby's birth weight. A woman of normal weight before pregnancy should gain about 30 pounds during pregnancy. Women who are underweight should gain more, about 34 pounds, and women who are obese can gain about 20. Women carrying twins should gain as much as 40 pounds. Recommended weight gains are based on your overall body mass, which is a calculation of weight for height (see Chapter 1 for recommended weight by height).

Women who are underweight during pregnancy are more likely to have small babies. Babies who have a low weight at birth (less than 5 1/2 pounds) have a more difficult time adjusting to life outside of the uterus. Proper nutrition and weight gain will help reduce the possibility of having an underweight baby. (Labor is not made easier because your baby is small or underweight. It is not appropriate to purposely gain less weight than is expected and required in order to have a smaller baby.)

If you gain weight as you should while you're pregnant, chances are that your baby will gain weight properly, too. You are not really "eating for two," though. The average woman will need to add only about 300 calories to her daily diet when she becomes pregnant. This is only an average, however, and your doctor will tell you whether you should eat more or less than this amount. For example, a teenager (who needs to fuel her own body's growth as well as her fetus's), an underweight woman, and a woman expecting twins should eat more than the average.

Women who are overweight can have problems during pregnancy, too. Still, it isn't a good idea to try to lose weight while you are pregnant, because you may deprive your baby of needed nutrients. It is best to try to lose weight before you are pregnant and then again after birth. Women who are overweight or who get very little exercise may be able to eat less than the average.

Eating snacks during the day is a good way to obtain needed nutrition and extra calories. It is best to pick snacks that have appropriate nutrients and are not high in concentrated sugars or fats. This usually means that candy, soda, and potato chips are of less value. Fruit, a slice of pizza, cereal, yogurt, and ice cream are healthier snacks.

You may feel more comfortable, especially during the later stages of pregnancy, eating small meals six times a day. To make these mini-meals, just divide the number of servings of the basic foods needed each day into smaller portions. Milk and a sandwich made with meat, chicken, fish, peanut butter, or cheese with lettuce and tomato make an excellent mini-meal. Other ideas are milk and fresh fruits, fruit juices, cheese and crackers, raw vegetables, and soup.

Iron

Women need a great deal more iron in their diet during pregnancy to support the fetus's growth and to produce extra blood in their bodies.

Where Does the Weight Go?

During pregnancy, most women should gain about 30 pounds. Changes to your body (increased size of the uterus, breast tissue, blood volume, and body fluid) account for the largest part of your weight gain. To support a pregnancy, your body must store nutrients and increase the volume of blood and other fluids it produces. One of the reasons for the extra fat is to prepare you to produce milk for breast-feeding.

7 pounds	Maternal stores (fat, protein, and other nutrients)
4 pounds	Increased fluid volume
4 pounds	Increased blood volume
2 pounds	Breast enlargement
2 pounds	Uterus
7 1/2 pounds	Baby
2 pounds	Amniotic fluid
1 1/2 pounds	Placenta (tissue connecting mother and baby that brings nourishment and takes away waste)

Iron is a mineral used by the body to make hemoglobin. Hemoglobin is the protein in the red blood cells that carries oxygen to the tissues and fetus. In most people, even after blood cells die, the body is able to save the iron to use in making more hemoglobin. Women, however, lose iron when they bleed during their menstrual periods. This makes it more difficult for women to eat the increased amounts of iron they need on a daily basis before pregnancy. Because few women have large enough stores of iron before they become pregnant, most have trouble getting the extra iron they need each day during pregnancy.

Eating foods rich in iron will provide some of the iron you need. However, many women find that they cannot get all the iron they need from their diet. Your doctor will probably recommend that you take an iron supplement to be sure that you are getting enough of this important mineral.

Folic Acid

During pregnancy, you need twice as much folic acid (400 μg) as you did before. Like iron, folic acid is used to make the extra blood you must produce. It is difficult to get all the extra folic acid you need just from your diet, so your doctor will probably have you take supplements of this vitamin, too.

Protein

Just as you need protein for the growth and repair of your muscles, so does your fetus. This extra need, plus your need to produce more blood, means that you should eat about 60 grams of protein each day. By choosing foods high in protein, you should be able to get the extra protein you and your fetus need.

Calcium and Phosphorus

Both of these minerals are used to make the fetus's bones. You need to get 1,200 mg of each every day—400 mg more than you needed before pregnancy if you're over 25. Drinking an extra quart of milk each day will give you the extra calcium that you need. Milk and other dairy products are the best sources of calcium, but other sources include sardines, salmon with bones, and greens (such as collard, kale, mustard, or turnip greens). If you cannot or do not eat milk products, you should mention this to your doctor. He or she may be able to suggest ways you can get the calcium you need.

Prenatal Vitamins

Except for iron, folic acid, and maybe calcium, you can usually get all the vitamins, minerals, and other nutrients you need during pregnancy by eating sensibly. In most cases, vitamin supplements are not necessary. However, if your doctor thinks that your diet may not be supplying all the nutrients you and your fetus need, he or she may prescribe a prenatal multivitamin and mineral supplement.

If your doctor prescribes prenatal vitamins, take them only as directed. It is especially important not to take more vitamins than your doctor directs. Large doses of vitamins can be dangerous. This is especially true with the fat-soluble vitamins A, D, E, and K. They can cause disease in the mother as well as abnormalities in the fetus. Too much vitamin C (a water-soluble vitamin) can also be dangerous.

Special Concerns

Most women will get all the additional nutrients they need during pregnancy if they eat a sensible diet and take vitamins as their doctor suggests. However, some women need more nutrients than a normal diet provides. You and your doctor will decide whether you fit into any of the following categories. If you do, your doctor can plan a special diet for your needs.

Teenagers

Teenagers are still growing themselves, so they need to provide for their own growth as well as the fetus's. Because their bones are still growing, they need 1,200 mg of calcium and 1,200 mg of phosphorus every day—400 mg more than a pregnant adult. They may be able to get these extra minerals from milk, or they may need to take supplements. Teenagers also need slightly more calories and protein than adults.

Women with Poor Nutrient Stores

If you have had three or more pregnancies within 2 years (including induced abortions and *miscarriages*), you have not had a chance to build up a store of nutrients in between pregnancies. A pregnancy is a big adjustment for your body. It is a good idea to let your body rest for at least a few months in between pregnancies. If you have previously had an abortion, a complicated pregnancy, or a low-birth-weight infant, or if you are underweight, your nutrient stores may be poor. Talk to your doctor about what extra nutrients you need and how to get them.

Special Diets

If you follow a special diet, you may not be getting all the nutrients you need. A vegetarian diet that includes milk, cheese, cereals, nuts, and seeds in addition to vegetables and fruits can be an adequate diet for a pregnant woman. If you eat a vegetarian diet, however, it must be planned carefully. A vegetarian diet that does not include milk does not supply all the nutrients a pregnant woman needs. If you are on a vegetarian diet, discuss food choices with your doctor, nutritionist, or dietitian. You may need to take supplements to get all the nutrients your body needs.

During pregnancy, some women feel an urge to eat nonfood items such as laundry starch or clay. This is called *pica*, and can be very common in some cultures. If you feel this urge, resist it and tell your doctor.

Women Who Smoke, Drink, or Use Drugs

Heavy smokers (women who smoke more than 11 cigarettes a day), women who take illegal drugs, and women who drink alcohol daily often have serious problems with nutrition as well as other complications in pregnancy. Their habit may prevent them from buying and eating healthy foods, or it may decrease their appetite for healthy foods. There is no better time than when you are pregnant to quit or cut down on dangerous habits such as smoking, drinking, and using drugs. Your doctor may be able to give you helpful suggestions on how to quit. If necessary, he or she can prescribe vitamin supplements for you.

Women with Certain Diseases

Some women have diseases that are long lasting and can cause problems with nutrition. The medication used to treat the disorder may affect the way in which food is absorbed by the body. Some diseases may require special diets that may make it hard for you to get all the nutrients you need. Be sure your doctor knows about any disease you have that could affect your nutrition. He or she may be able to change your medication, recommend a different diet, or take other steps to help you get the nutrients you need.

Questions to Consider...

- Am I eating enough to get the vitamins, nutrients, and calories I need during pregnancy?
- How much weight should I gain during pregnancy?
- Should I take a vitamin–mineral supplement?
- Do I need to make any special adjustments to my diet?

Chapter 9

Changes During Pregnancy

As your fetus grows, your uterus increases to about 1,000 times its original size. This amount of growth, centered in one area, affects other parts of your body. Many of the changes in your body that occur during pregnancy are triggered by hormones (substances produced by the body to control the functions of various organs) that nurture the fetus and prepare for childbirth. These changes have a physical and emotional impact and may cause discomforts. Some may occur only in the early weeks of pregnancy. Others may occur only as you get closer to the end of your pregnancy. Still others may appear early, then go away, only to return again later. This is normal and usually does not mean that anything is wrong. Every woman's pregnancy is unique, as are her responses to it. Share your concerns, discomforts, and questions with your doctor, who may be able to suggest things you can do to make yourself feel more comfortable.

Physical Changes

Backache

Backache is one of the most common complaints during pregnancy. It is usually caused by the strain put on the back muscles by your growing uterus and by changes in your posture. Here are some suggestions to help lessen back pain:

- Wear low-heeled (but not flat) shoes.
- Avoid lifting heavy objects or children.
- Do not bend over from the waist to pick things up—squat down, bending your knees and keeping your back straight.
- Place one foot on a stool or box when you have to stand for long periods.

- Arrange things at home and at work at a comfortable level, so that you don't have to bend or stretch too much.
- Check that your bed is firm enough. If it is too soft, placing a board between the mattress and box spring (have someone help you) can be helpful.
- Sleep on your side with one knee bent and your upper leg supported on a pillow.
- Apply heat, cold, or pressure to the painful area.
- Do special exercises—ask your doctor or nurse for specific instructions.

Breast Changes

Starting early in pregnancy, your breasts undergo many changes to prepare for breast-feeding your baby. In fact, changes to your breasts may be one of the first signs that you are pregnant. By 6–8 weeks of pregnancy, your breasts will be noticeably larger. This is because the fat layer of your breasts is thickening, and the number of milk glands is increasing.

Your breasts will continue to grow in size and weight throughout the first *trimester*. Changes in breast size may be more obvious in women with small breasts and less obvious in women with large breasts. Your breasts will feel firm and tender. As your breasts grow, wearing a good bra that fits well will provide you with support. To fuel the growth of your breasts, their blood supply increases, and the veins close to the surface become larger and more noticeable. You may feel some tingling, or your breasts may be sensitive to touch.

Also early in pregnancy, your nipples and *areolas* (the darker skin around your nipples) will darken. Your nipples may project out more now. This helps your baby firmly latch on to your breast if you breast-feed. Your areolas also grow larger. On the surface of the areolas are small glands called Montgomery tubercles. They produce an oily substance that helps protect the nipple from cracking or drying out. The Montgomery tubercles now become raised and bumpy.

If you plan to breast-feed, you may want to prepare your nipples. To toughen the area where

During pregnancy (top), the fat layer of your breasts thickens and the number of milk glands increases, making them larger than before pregnancy (bottom).

Milk glands

Fat

A woman with retracted nipples (top) can prepare for breast-feeding by doing exercises (bottom).

your baby will suck, you can expose your breasts to air, wear a nursing bra with the flaps down, or gently rub your nipples with a washcloth. Soaps or creams should not be used.

Some women's nipples do not project out but sink inward (***retracted nipple***). If you have retracted nipples and you plan to breast-feed, your doctor may recommend that you try massaging the nipples so they protrude more. You can also gently pull on either side of the areola with your forefingers. In time, this will also cause the nipple to stick out.

By about 12–14 weeks of pregnancy, your breasts may begin producing ***colostrum***, the fluid that will feed your baby for his or her first few days before your milk comes in. This doesn't happen in every woman, so don't be concerned if you don't produce colostrum before delivery. Colostrum contains water, proteins, minerals, and ***antibodies*** that protect your baby from disease. Early in pregnancy, the colostrum will probably be thick and yellow, but toward the end of pregnancy, it will become pale and nearly colorless. Colostrum may leak from your breasts by itself or if you massage your breasts. It also tends to leak out during times of sexual excitement.

Breathing Problems

As the fetus grows inside your uterus, the uterus expands and takes up more room in your abdomen. In the third trimester, by about 31–34 weeks of pregnancy, the uterus has grown so large that it presses the digestive organs and the diaphragm (a flat, strong muscle that aids in breathing) up toward the lungs. Because the lungs do not have as much room to expand as before, you may find you are short of breath. Even if you feel you are not getting enough air, you need not worry about the fetus. It will get all the oxygen it needs.

A few weeks before you give birth, the fetus's head will move down in the uterus, or "drop," and press against the cervix. This usually happens between 36–38 weeks of pregnancy in women who have not been pregnant before, but in women who have already been pregnant, it may not happen until the beginning of labor. When the fetus drops, you will find it easier to breathe, because the uterus will not be pressing as much on your other organs.

If being short of breath makes you uncomfortable, here are some ideas to try:

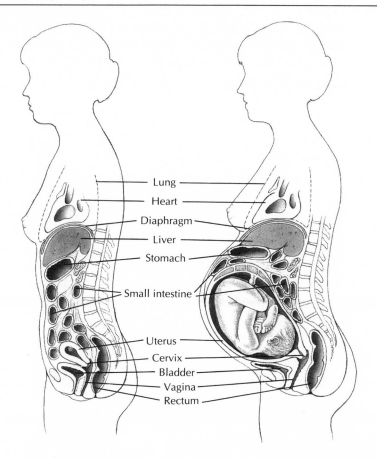

As the uterus grows from the beginning (left) *toward the end of pregnancy* (right)*, it takes up more room in your abdomen, pressing the digestive organs and diaphragm up toward the lungs.*

- Take life a little more slowly, so your heart and lungs don't have to work so hard.
- Sit up straight.
- Sleep propped up.
- Ask your doctor or a childbirth educator about breathing exercises to help you breathe more deeply.

Constipation

At least half of all pregnant women seem to have problems with constipation. One reason for this may be changes in hormones that slow the movement of food through the digestive tract. During the last part of pregnancy, pressure on your rectum from your uterus may add to the problem. Here are some suggestions that may help:

- Drink plenty of liquids—at least eight glasses each day, including fruit juices such as prune juice.
- Eat food high in fiber, such as raw fruits and vegetables and bran cereals.
- Exercise daily—just walking is fine.

Cramps

In the last 3 months of pregnancy, you may find that you have leg cramps. Although it was once thought that cramps were caused by a problem with the amount of calcium in your diet, this is no longer thought to be true. Stretching your legs before going to bed can help relieve cramps, but avoid pointing your toes when stretching or exercising.

Fatigue

You may feel tired often during pregnancy—especially during the first and last 3 months. The remedy for fatigue relies on common sense: get enough exercise and rest (including naps) and eat a well-balanced diet.

Frequent Urination

There is usually a desire to urinate frequently during the first 3 months of pregnancy. It is mainly caused by the pressure of the growing uterus on the bladder, the organ in which urine is stored. Even though your bladder may be nearly empty, this pressure produces the same kind of sensation as when the bladder is full of urine.

Kegel Exercises

Kegel exercises, or perineal exercises, are used to strengthen the muscles that surround the openings of the urethra, vagina, and anus. Your doctor or nurse can help you learn to perform these exercises. If you contract these muscles for about 3 seconds, 12–15 times in a row, at least six times a day, in time you will begin to notice some improvement in your ability to hold your urine.

As your uterus grows and rises higher into your abdomen, the symptoms may disappear. In the last month or so, though, urinary frequency may return as the fetus drops into the pelvis and again presses against the bladder. Especially toward the end of pregnancy, you may find that the need to urinate wakes you up several times during the night. If the pressure of the uterus on the bladder causes you to leak some urine, there are special exercises called Kegel exercises that can help strengthen the muscles around the urethra (the tube that carries urine from the bladder out of the body). If you have pain when you urinate or if you often feel you need to urinate right away, you should talk to your doctor. You could have an infection.

Groin or Lower Abdominal Pain

As the uterus grows, the round ligaments (bands of fibrous tissue along both sides of the uterus) that support it are pulled and stretched. You may occasionally feel this as either sharp pains in your abdomen, usually on the side, or a dull ache. The pains are most common between 18–24 weeks. To help prevent these pains, avoid quick changes of position, especially when you are turning at the waist. When you do feel a pain, bend toward it to relieve it. Resting and changing your position also seem to help.

Hemorrhoids

Very often pregnant women who are constipated also have hemorrhoids. Hemorrhoids are varicose (or swollen) veins of the rectum. They are often painful. Straining during bowel movements and having very hard stools may increase the severity of hemorrhoids and sometimes may cause them to protrude from the rectum.

Do not take drugstore cures while you are pregnant without first checking with your doctor. Several things can help give relief or avoid the problem in the first place:

- Avoid constipation.
- Eat a high-fiber diet.
- Drink plenty of liquids.
- Exercise.

Indigestion

Indigestion is commonly called heartburn, but it does not mean that anything is wrong with your heart. It is a burning sensation that is first felt in the stomach and seems to rise up into the throat. It occurs when digested food from your stomach, which contains acid, is pushed up into your esophagus (the tube leading from the throat to the stomach). Because liquids are foods and take up space in your stomach, they can also contribute to the problem.

Changes that take place in your body during pregnancy may worsen indigestion. Changes in your hormone levels slow digestion and relax the muscle that keeps the digested food and acids in your stomach, preventing it from entering the esophagus. In addition, your growing uterus presses up on your stomach.

To help relieve heartburn, try the following:

- Eat five or six small meals a day instead of two or three large ones.
- Avoid foods that cause gas, such as spicy or greasy foods.
- Sit up while eating.
- Wait an hour after eating before lying down and do not eat before bedtime.
- Wait 2 hours after eating before exercising.

Do not take any medications unless you first check with your doctor. This includes antacids and baking soda.

Insomnia

This problem is especially evident in the last months of pregnancy, when your abdomen has grown so large that a comfortable position can be hard to find. Several remedies can help you to get the rest you need:

- A warm bath at bedtime
- Relaxation techniques learned in childbirth classes
- Lying on your side with a pillow supporting your abdomen and another between your legs
- Short periods of rest during the day

Nausea and Vomiting

Most often caused by changes in hormones, nausea and vomiting are common complaints during the first 3 months of pregnancy. Nausea and vomiting sometimes return late in pregnancy. They are usually called morning sickness, but they can occur any time during the day, especially when the stomach is empty. There are some things you can do to feel more comfortable:

- Arise slowly when you wake up and sit on the side of the bed for a few minutes.
- Eat dry toast, crackers, a peeled apple, or a plain potato (peeled and cooked).
- Eat five or six small meals each day—try to avoid having your stomach completely empty.
- Avoid unpleasant odors when possible.
- Avoid drinking citrus juice, water, milk, coffee, and tea.

If nausea or vomiting becomes severe, notify your doctor. Always check with your doctor before taking any medication.

Numbness and Tingling

As the uterus increases in size and rests on certain nerves, numbness and tingling in the legs, toes, and sometimes in the arms may occur. This is usually not serious and will go away after the baby is born.

Skin Changes

The different amounts of hormones in your body often contribute to some normal changes on certain areas of your skin. Some women notice brownish, uneven blotches around the eyes and over the nose and cheekbones. This is called *chloasma*. These marks usually disappear or fade after delivery, when hormone levels go back to normal. Being in the sunlight tends to increase these skin changes.

Many women notice the darkening of a line running from the top to the bottom of the abdomen. This is called the *linea nigra*. Others may notice streaks or stretch marks on the abdomen and breasts as they grow during pregnancy. This is caused by the skin tissue stretching to support the extra weight. There is no way to prevent stretch marks, but they will slowly fade after pregnancy.

Swelling

A certain amount of swelling (called *edema*) seems to be normal during pregnancy. It occurs most often in the legs, and usually disappears in the morning. Swelling can begin during the last few months of pregnancy, and it may occur more often in the summer. Let your doctor know if you have swelling in your hands or face, because this may mean that there is another problem. Never take medicines for swelling unless your doctor has prescribed them. You can help the swelling in your legs go down by trying these suggestions:

- Elevate your legs when possible.
- Rest in bed on your side, preferably your left side.
- Do not wear anything that binds your legs, such as tight garters or bands around stockings or socks.
- Exercise regularly, especially walking, swimming, or riding an exercise bike.
- Wear support pantyhose or stockings.

Varicose Veins

Varicose, or swollen, veins appear most often in the legs but can also appear near the vulva and vagina. They are caused by pressure from the weight of your uterus on your veins and frequently develop if you must stand or sit for long periods of time. This condition is usually not serious but can be uncomfortable and may cause aching, sore legs. Some of these suggestions may help:

- Elevate your legs when possible.
- Lie on the floor with your legs raised on a small footstool or several pillows. Tuck a pillow under one hip so that you are not absolutely flat on the floor.
- If your job requires much sitting, stand up and move around frequently to help your circulation.
- Try not to stand for long periods of time.
- Do not wear anything that binds your legs, such as tight garters or bands around stockings or socks.
- Wear support stockings, or your doctor can recommend special elastic stockings.

Emotional Changes

Pregnancy is a time of not only physical changes but also emotional changes. Although many women feel very good during pregnancy, the increase of hormones that enable a woman's body to maintain and support the pregnancy may also result in mood swings, especially during the first 3 months. Extreme tiredness in early and late pregnancy may also make you feel irritable or depressed. Regular periods of rest and relaxation will help your emotional as well as physical well-being.

Mood Swings

Perhaps the worst thing about mood swings is that they are unpredictable. A minor problem may not bother you one day and may have you in tears the next. Not knowing how you will react to a situation makes it hard on you, your family, and your friends. These unpredictable changes are often caused by the changes in your levels of hormones. These changes are not something you can control, so don't blame yourself if you are often teary or short-tempered.

The hormones that are needed to support your pregnancy form a complex system: levels of some hormones are rising, while levels of others are falling. These changes are needed to bring about all the different stages of your pregnancy. When hormones control so many functions in the body, it makes sense that constantly changing levels would affect you.

Although pregnancy is mostly a happy time, you may feel sad or worried now and then. These feelings are normal and are caused partly by the changes in your hormone levels. Fatigue can also cause or worsen feelings of sadness. Especially during the last few weeks of pregnancy, you may feel tired often. The newness of being pregnant has worn off, and the extra weight you are carrying may make you feel heavy and slow. These feelings will usually pass quickly after delivery.

Anxiety

Pregnant women and their partners often have many fears and worries about the pregnancy, labor and delivery, the effect of a child on their lives, and whether they will be good parents. Usually there is nothing to worry about, but these feelings may prompt you to make decisions and take actions that will help things go more smoothly.

Many parents-to-be worry that their child will not be normal. By far, most children are born healthy. You know that you can take steps to help ensure a healthy child. These include eating right; resting and exercising; avoiding drugs, alcohol, and a high-risk sexual life style; and receiving early and regular prenatal care. You can also take advantage of any tests your doctor recommends that can show the health of the fetus.

Women also are often anxious about labor and delivery, especially if they have not given birth before. Learning what to expect can be a big help. You may fear the pain and think that you won't be able to stand it. You can prepare for labor and the birth of your child by learning about methods that can help relieve pain. These methods for breathing and relaxing are taught in childbirth preparation classes. Different kinds of pain medication also can help you during labor and birth. Even if you hadn't planned on using pain medication, don't feel as though you have failed if you need it. You cannot be a good participant in the birth of your baby if you are in a great deal of pain. Medication can help ease the pain enough so that you can do your part as you practiced.

Although all the instruction you've received about giving birth may have convinced you otherwise, having a baby is a natural event. There are no grades given for having a baby. If you plan to use childbirth preparation techniques, you may fear that you will forget them. Practice will make them second nature.

If your labor is very long or if the size or position of your fetus presents a problem, you may need some help in childbirth. If instruments such as *forceps* are used, or if your doctor decides you need to deliver by a cesarean birth instead of vaginally, do not think that you have failed. Sometimes things don't go according to plan. You and your partner will want to be flexible and do what is best for you and the baby, even if it hasn't been rehearsed ahead of time.

Every parent is new to parenthood at some time and must learn how to care for, feed, and bathe a baby. If this is your first child, usually a nurse or someone at the hospital will be able to help you learn the basics about caring for the baby before you go home. Once you're home, your family and friends will probably also give you their own advice.

There are as many different ways of raising a baby as there are children. You will find the one that is right for you. Talking to other mothers can help relieve you of some fears and give you practical tips you can use. There are also a number of good books and classes on child care. Your pediatrician, the baby's doctor, may be able to recommend some for you.

Having a baby will mean big changes in your life. It doesn't mean, however, that you will be trapped or that the baby will take over your lives. You and your partner can still enjoy activities you shared before you became pregnant, and can now alter them to include your baby.

Body Image

When you are pregnant, your body undergoes nearly a total remaking—all the more amazing because of how fast it happens. It can be hard for your mind to keep up with your body's changes. As your breasts enlarge, your waistline begins disappearing, and your abdomen grows larger, you may have very mixed feelings. On the one hand, this change is an exciting, very visible reminder of the new life growing inside you. There will probably be days, though, when you'll just feel fat and wonder if you'll ever have your old body back. It is normal to have mixed feelings about the changes in your body.

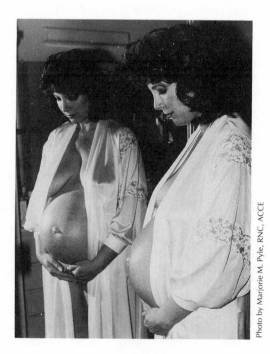

Photo by Marjorie M. Pyle, RNC, ACCE

Exercise may help you feel better about how you look and, after delivery, can help you get back in shape.

Your Partner

Both you and your partner will have many adjustments to make throughout your pregnancy. Your old roles are changing, and you need to work to adapt to your new roles. You both may spend much of your time thinking about the baby, and you need to remember to make time for each other. Try to be understanding of each other. Pregnancy is a special time for a couple, but it can also cause stress and strains in your relationship because so much is changing. Being in a supportive relationship eases the course of pregnancy and the move into parenthood.

Because all the physical changes of pregnancy are happening to you, it is easy to forget that your partner is a part of the pregnancy, too. He is making his own adjustments, getting ready to be a father. Make a special effort to include him in things. Don't shut him out. Let him be a part of your pregnancy plans. He should attend childbirth classes with you and join you in exercising, buying clothes for the baby, and getting the baby's space ready.

Your sexual feelings about each other may also change. It is a good idea to talk to each other, so that you understand how your partner is feeling and so that he understands your concerns. Talking

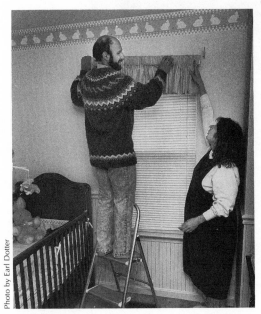

Photo by Earl Dotter

can bring you closer and help avoid hurt feelings and loneliness due to misunderstandings. Some couples find that pregnancy brings them together and that they feel closer than ever.

Because of your increased hormone levels and the fact that your body may be more sensitive to touch, you may be more easily aroused. Many men and women find a pregnant woman's larger breasts and rounded abdomen very sensuous. Other couples find that it is harder to enjoy sex now. Especially during the first and third trimesters, when you are more likely to feel nauseated and tired, sex may seem like a big bother. Your thoughts may focus on the baby, and your sexual feelings may be pushed aside. You or your partner may worry about injuring the baby if you have sex. In most cases, this will not happen, but for more guidelines, see "Sex," Chapter 7, and ask your doctor.

Questions to Consider...

- What can I do to relieve the discomforts of pregnancy?
- What if morning sickness doesn't go away or becomes very severe?
- Do I need to do anything to prepare my breasts for breast-feeding?
- Is it all right to take any over-the-counter medications if I feel really uncomfortable?
- If I develop varicose veins or hemorrhoids, will they go away after the baby is born?
- Are there ways in which my partner can become more involved in the pregnancy?

Chapter 10

Special Care Pregnancies

Pregnancy puts new demands on a woman's body. It can alter the course of some medical conditions a woman may have before pregnancy, and some conditions can affect the course of pregnancy. A woman with such a medical condition can have a healthy baby. An extra effort will be required, however, so that the woman's general health and her pregnancy can be followed more closely.

If you have a condition that could complicate your pregnancy, your doctor may order additional tests and ask you to make extra prenatal visits or attend special clinics. You may need to stay in the hospital or to monitor your condition yourself at home. Your doctor may work with a team of experts to provide any special care you may need.

High Blood Pressure

Hypertension, or high blood pressure, occurs when the pressure of the blood in the arteries reaches levels that are greater than normal. This condition can be preexisting (before pregnancy) and chronic (long-term), or it can arise during pregnancy. High blood pressure that arises during pregnancy can be a sign of a condition called *preeclampsia* (also known as toxemia). These two conditions—chronic high blood pressure and preeclampsia—affect pregnancy and its outcome in different ways. Depending on how severe these conditions are, both the mother and fetus can be affected.

Heart

Arter

Vein

The heart pumps blood rich in oxygen through the arteries (light blood vessels) *to all parts of the body. Blood returns to the heart through the veins* (dark blood vessels). *If a blood pressure reading is 110/80, 110 is the pressure in the arteries when the heart is contracting, or the systolic pressure. The lower number, 80, is the pressure in the arteries when the heart is relaxed, or the diastolic pressure.*

Measuring Blood Pressure

Blood pressure is checked with a stethoscope and an instrument made of an inflatable cuff and a pressure gauge (sphygmomanometer). A blood pressure reading is made up of two numbers separated by a slash, for example, 110/80. (You may hear this referred to as "110 over 80.") The first number is the pressure in the arteries when the heart contracts. This is called the systolic pressure. The second number is the pressure in the arteries when the heart is relaxed between contractions. This is the diastolic pressure.

Blood pressure changes often during the day. It can rise if you are excited or if you exercise. It usually falls when you are resting. These temporary changes in blood pressure that occur in response to some activity or event are normal. It is only when a person's blood pressure stays high for some time that it requires attention.

Because of the normal ups and downs in blood pressure, if your doctor finds one high reading, he or she will want to see whether it is your normal level by taking another reading. Your normal blood pressure can be an average of several readings taken at rest.

Blood pressure varies from person to person, so everyone's blood pressure is different. In nonpregnant adults, readings less than 130/80 are usually normal, and become abnormal when pressures reach above 140/90.

Some blood pressure levels that may seem normal could be too high in a pregnant woman. For instance, a reading of 120/85 would be considered too high for a pregnant woman whose normal reading was 90/70. As a rule, any increase of 30 or more in the systolic reading or 15 or more in the diastolic reading can be a sign of high blood pressure in pregnancy.

Warning Signs and Symptoms of High Blood Pressure

These signs and symptoms are sometimes linked to high blood pressure in pregnancy and should warn you to have your blood pressure checked:

- Severe and constant headaches
- Swelling (*edema*), especially of the face
- Dizziness
- Blurred vision or spots in front of the eyes
- Sudden weight gain of more than about 1 pound a day

It is normal for blood pressure to drop slightly during the middle part of pregnancy and then return to prepregnancy levels during the latter part of pregnancy. Because of these changes, it is important to have your blood pressure measured before pregnancy or in early pregnancy so your doctor will know what is normal for you. As a part of prenatal care, a woman's blood pressure is checked at each visit.

Chronic High Blood Pressure

High blood pressure can be present when a woman becomes pregnant. Diet, life style, and heredity contribute to chronic high blood pressure. Over the course of her life, a woman with untreated high blood pressure is more likely to have a heart attack or stroke. She is also at higher risk for having problems during pregnancy. These include having a baby that is too small or separation of the *placenta* from the wall of the uterus before the fetus is born.

Before you get pregnant, chronic hypertension should be brought under control with diet, weight loss, and possibly medication. During pregnancy, regular checkups are important to detect any changes in your condition that may signal a problem.

Preeclampsia

High blood pressure that occurs for the first time in the second half of pregnancy along with protein in the urine and, usually, fluid retention is called preeclampsia. It affects about 7 out of every 100 women who become pregnant. It is not known what causes preeclampsia, although women who have chronic high blood pressure are more likely to develop it. Most women with preeclampsia, however, have never had high blood pressure before. Preeclampsia usually occurs with first pregnancies and often does not recur in later pregnancies except in women who have chronic hypertension or other diseases affecting the blood vessels. With preeclampsia, blood pressure returns to normal levels after pregnancy, whereas chronic hypertension remains after delivery.

The blood vessels in the uterus supply blood to the placenta, through which the fetus is nourished and given oxygen. When a woman has preeclampsia, the blood flow through these vessels is reduced. The severity of the condition and the time in pregnancy when it occurs determines the degree of risk to the fetus.

When blood pressure increases during pregnancy, your doctor

may recommend bed rest. Frequently, the blood pressure will improve or return to normal with rest. When resting, the woman may be advised to lie on her side—this position improves the flow of blood to the uterus and kidneys. Some doctors hospitalize women as soon as there is a slight increase in blood pressure; others wait until there is evidence that bed rest at home has not helped to reduce blood pressure.

Preeclampsia occurs in degrees, from mild to severe, and can gradually worsen or improve. If preeclampsia is detected in mild stages and controlled by bed rest and medication, the effects on the baby can be reduced. The goal, all other factors permitting, is to allow the pregnancy to continue until the fetus is old enough to be born.

When preeclampsia occurs early and is severe, early delivery may be necessary. A premature baby is underweight and may have trouble breathing because the lungs are not fully developed. When preeclampsia is associated with chronic hypertension, the placenta can separate from the uterus and result in *stillbirth*. Preeclampsia can also be linked to poor fetal growth. Severe preeclampsia can be fatal to the mother, although this is very rare. The disease affects almost all of the mother's organs, such as the blood system, liver, kidneys, and brain. Convulsions can occur without warning with preeclampsia. When this occurs, the disease is called eclampsia. The treatment for very severe preeclampsia or eclampsia is to deliver the fetus, either by inducing labor or performing a cesarean birth.

Diabetes

Diabetes is a condition that occurs when there is a problem with the way the body makes or uses *insulin*. Insulin is a hormone that helps the body use *glucose*, a sugar that is the body's main source of fuel. When the body doesn't make enough insulin, or when the usual effect of insulin or glucose does not occur as it should, the level of glucose in the blood becomes too high because it is not being used by the body properly. Diabetes can be present before pregnancy or develop during pregnancy. With either type, insulin may be needed to control glucose levels.

Gestational Diabetes

Some women develop diabetes when they become pregnant. This is called gestational diabetes. It results from the effects of hormones made by the placenta during pregnancy. These hormones can alter the way in which insulin works. When abnormal glucose levels first develop during pregnancy, they can do so without symptoms. Usually, the glucose level returns to normal after delivery. Women who have gestational diabetes have a higher risk of developing diabetes again later in life, however.

Diabetes is more likely to occur during pregnancy in women who are age 30 and older, obese, have had problems such as stillbirth or a very large baby in a previous pregnancy, and have a family history of diabetes. If one or more of these risk factors exist, your doctor may decide to test you for diabetes during pregnancy. This safe and simple test is usually done about two-thirds of the way through your pregnancy. A sample of blood is taken exactly 1 hour after you drink a special sugar solution. If the blood glucose level is high, a similar but longer test, usually taking 3 hours, will be done. This is called a glucose tolerance test.

Women who have uncomplicated gestational diabetes may not need insulin; instead, they can control their blood glucose levels by eating a special diet. In this case, blood glucose levels usually are not tested daily. When insulin is used to control gestational diabetes, the diet and the insulin dose must be regulated to prevent the harmful effects of high and low blood glucose levels.

If risks are not controlled, the risk of having a large baby (*macrosomia*) increases. Large babies have difficulty at birth, particularly in delivery of the shoulders. Special testing may be necessary to evaluate the fetus before it is born.

With gestational diabetes, blood glucose levels usually return to normal after birth, but diabetes can recur. You may have another test several months after delivery to make sure you are no longer diabetic. If you are overweight, you and your doctor will set up a balanced program of diet and exercise for you to follow after delivery. This may reduce the risk of problems in later pregnancies and may help lower the risk of developing diabetes later in life.

Preexisting Diabetes

About 1% of women of childbearing age have diabetes. At one time, diabetes posed a major health risk to the mother and fetus during pregnancy. Today, however, more is known about diabetes and how to control it, so pregnancy is safer for most diabetic women.

The outlook for diabetic pregnancies gets better each day. It has improved to the point where the risks for a diabetic pregnancy are almost as low as those for a normal uncomplicated pregnancy. The degree of risk posed by diabetes is directly related to how well the condition is controlled before and during pregnancy. Ideally, the diabetes should be diagnosed and brought under control before pregnancy, and then carefully monitored to keep blood glucose levels as normal as possible. With careful planning, control of diabetes, and expert care, the chances for a successful pregnancy—a healthy baby and mother—are very good.

Risks. Although there is no cure for diabetes, it can be effectively treated, and there is less risk to the fetus when the condition is under control before and during pregnancy. Woman who have diabetes when they become pregnant should receive early care to help lower these risks:

- Preeclampsia, or high blood pressure during pregnancy, can require the baby to be delivered early or can slow its growth while in the uterus.
- *Hydramnios* (too much *amniotic fluid* in the sac surrounding the fetus) can make it difficult for the mother to breathe and may also result in premature labor and delivery.
- Macrosomia (a larger-than-normal baby) occurs in less severe cases and can make delivery difficult.
- Birth defects are more common in babies of diabetic mothers, especially if the diabetes is not well controlled.
- *Miscarriage* occurs more often in diabetic women, especially if the condition is not under control.
- *Respiratory distress syndrome* may affect the baby's ability to breathe because the lungs are not fully developed.
- Stillbirth, although uncommon, also occurs more often in babies of diabetic mothers.

Controlling Diabetes. Your diet is an important way to control your glucose levels. The number of calories in your diet will depend on both your weight and the stage of pregnancy. Your doctor may adjust your diet from time to time to improve blood glucose control or to meet the needs of the growing fetus. Usually the diet consists of special meals and snacks spread throughout the day. A bedtime snack helps to maintain blood glucose levels during the night.

Regular exercise also plays an important role in the control of diabetes. It reduces the amount of insulin needed to maintain normal blood glucose levels. The amount of exercise that is right for each

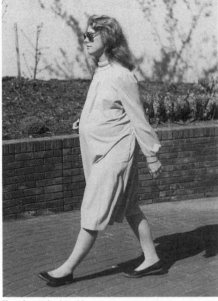

Photo by Michael Dodd

woman varies. Among other things, it depends on the stage of pregnancy.

Some diabetics need to take insulin to keep their blood glucose at a normal level. Insulin can be taken by injection only. It does not cross the placenta, so it does not affect the fetus directly. The amount of insulin needed to control blood glucose levels throughout the day varies from woman to woman and depends on many factors. In many cases, insulin must be taken at least twice a day during pregnancy. Usually the need for insulin increases throughout the pregnancy, leveling off near the end. This means that the insulin dose needs to be adjusted from time to time for good control of blood glucose levels. This is where home monitoring of blood glucose levels plays an important role.

If you have diabetes that must be controlled with insulin, you will need to monitor your blood glucose on a day-to-day basis to keep it at a normal level as much of the time as possible. There are a number of ways to do this, all of which are safe and simple to use. You and your doctor will decide together on the best method or combination of methods for you.

Blood glucose meters or colored strips can be used to measure blood glucose levels at home. In either method, a simple device is used to obtain a small drop of blood, usually from the tip of the finger. The blood glucose level is then read with the meter or strip. Both of these methods provide reliable results when used properly.

Because the blood glucose level normally changes throughout the day, it usually must be checked several times a day. Your doctor will advise you as to how often you will need to check your blood glucose.

When diabetes is not controlled and the body cannot use glucose for energy, it resorts to burning fat. Certain substances called ketones

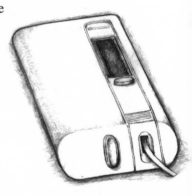

Glucose meters or strips can be used to measure glucose levels in blood.

produced as a result of burning the fat may be found in the urine. Ketones in the urine can be a sign of ketoacidosis, a serious complication of uncontrolled diabetes that can cause stillbirth.

Special Care for Diabetics. A woman with diabetes usually needs to have certain tests done more often in her pregnancy. These tests can help the doctor identify problems that may occur early and take steps to correct them. One test measures hemoglobin A1C, a substance in the mother's blood. When levels are higher than normal, they indicate that the control of the body's glucose use has been poor for a number of weeks. Other tests, such as **ultrasound**, **amniocentesis**, and fetal monitoring, are used to assess the present status and growth of the fetus. These tests are especially important if the baby must be delivered early.

Early in your pregnancy, you may need to stay briefly in a hospital so that your blood glucose levels can be controlled and your general health can be assessed. Additional hospital stays may be needed, depending on your blood glucose levels and any other health problems you may be having. The trend has been to reduce the length of these hospital stays.

At one time, almost all women with diabetes had cesarean births because the potential problems associated with diabetic pregnancy could be made worse by the added stress of labor and vaginal delivery. Today, however, with special tests and monitoring methods, most women with diabetes are able to give birth safely through the vagina.

Heart Disease

Women who have heart disease during their reproductive years may have either rheumatic heart disease or congenital heart disease. Because of advances in preventing rheumatic heart disease, it is a less common problem in pregnancy. Women with congenital heart disease are born with an anatomic defect in the heart. The nature and severity of this defect determine whether they may be at risk of having problems during pregnancy.

Ideally, heart disease should be diagnosed before conception. Once the condition is diagnosed, all possible steps can be taken to correct it. Counseling also can be provided about the impact of the disease on the pregnancy and vice versa. If you have serious cardiac disease, your doctor will work in a team approach with a cardiologist to manage your care throughout the pregnancy.

Pregnancy increases the work the heart has to do, and labor and delivery place added stress on the heart. The amount of blood the heart pumps increases by up to 40% during pregnancy. Physical activity may need to be limited so that the demand on the heart is lessened. Your doctor will prescribe a routine of rest and possibly medications.

During labor, contractions increase the heart's work load, as do the pain and anxiety that go along with them. In spite of this, when obstetric conditions permit, vaginal delivery is preferred over cesarean birth because it causes less stress to the heart. *Anesthesia* may be given during labor to reduce pain and anxiety.

Women with heart disease are more likely to deliver prematurely, and their babies are often smaller than they should be. The babies of mothers who have congenital heart disease have a 4–5% chance of having the disease as well, although it may not be serious or life-threatening. New techniques for diagnosing heart disease in the fetus have improved the accuracy of this diagnosis and make it possible to plan for special care.

Lung Disorders

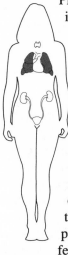

Pregnancy causes a number of changes in a woman's breathing patterns. Due to the growing uterus, the shape of the chest cavity is changed. It is quite common for a pregnant woman to feel short of breath (for hints on ways to feel more comfortable when you are short of breath, see "Physical Changes," Chapter 9). There are certain lung disorders, however, that may cause changes beyond this common shortness of breath.

Asthma, a lung disorder that causes wheezing and breathing problems, is one of the more common problems. It has not been shown to worsen or improve during pregnancy, but it could pose problems if the fetus does not get enough oxygen. Most women with asthma can go safely through a pregnancy, continuing to use their inhalers or prescribed medicines to help them breathe and supply the fetus with enough oxygen. Most of the medicines used for asthma are safe during pregnancy, except those containing iodine or tetracycline. Therefore, your doctor needs to know which medicines you take. Women with severe asthma must have their problem carefully controlled and be watched closely, because their asthma attacks will probably continue during pregnancy.

Pneumonia is an infection in the lungs that may be more serious in pregnancy than it is at other times. It may result in the mother and fetus getting less oxygen, and so it should be diagnosed and treated promptly. A chest X-ray is usually an important step in finding pneumonia. The technician who takes the X-ray may place a lead apron on your abdomen to shield the fetus. This type of X-ray has not been shown to cause any harm to the fetus (see "Harmful Agents," Chapter 7). A pregnant woman with pneumonia is often hospitalized to receive *antibiotics*, many of which are safe for the mother and fetus.

Renal Disease

During pregnancy, more blood flows to the kidneys as they work harder to filter waste products faster to take care of the needs of both the woman and her fetus. If a woman's kidneys are weakened from a previous disease or do not work properly, it could have an effect on her pregnancy. With proper medical treatment, however, risks usually can be reduced. Some disorders that affect the kidney are linked with high blood pressure. If the blood pressure can be controlled, the risk of problems during pregnancy is reduced.

Kidney disease can usually be diagnosed on the basis of your medical history, physical exam, and blood and urine tests. Protein in the urine may be a sign of kidney disease. It can be caused by diseases that interfere with kidney function. Urinary tract infections and high blood pressure in a previous pregnancy also are signs that require further evaluation.

Epilepsy

Women with epilepsy or seizures (convulsions) can have safe pregnancies. Seizures may be minor problems involving muscle control or major attacks involving loss of control of bladder or bowel function and blackout spells. Usually women with seizures take medicines prescribed to control or prevent repeated seizures.

A woman with epilepsy has a risk two to three times higher than normal of having a baby with a birth defect, especially cleft lip and palate or heart defects. The reason for the higher risk is not clear. It is known, however, that some of the drugs taken to control seizures can cause birth defects. However, a seizure or repeated seizures could be harmful to the mother or fetus as well. Therefore, a woman with epilepsy should discuss continued drug use with her doctor. Sometimes the medication can be changed before or during pregnancy to reduce the risks.

Autoimmune Disorders

The autoimmune disorders are a group of diseases in which the body's immune system, which is designed to protect it, goes awry, attacking and injuring the body's own tissues. The injury may be in a specific organ, such as the kidney, or in various parts of the body.

Most autoimmune diseases are chronic conditions for which there is no cure. It is not always known what causes them. Their symptoms can disappear for a time and then recur with little warning or without apparent reason. The effects on pregnancy depend on the type of disorder.

Many of the autoimmune diseases have overlapping signs and symptoms, making them difficult to diagnose. Your doctor may work with a specialist in planning care for your pregnancy.

Systemic Lupus Erythematosus

Systemic lupus erythematosus (SLE) is a disease that can affect the entire body, including skin, joints, kidneys, and the nervous system. Its results can range from minor skin sores to a serious fatal condition in which the kidneys fail and the nervous system, heart, and blood are affected.

SLE tends to occur in young women during their childbearing years. It does not appear to affect fertility, but it increases the risks of miscarriage, premature deliveries, and stillbirth. A baby of a woman with SLE can be born with a heart defect.

In approximately 30% of women with SLE, the disease becomes more severe during pregnancy, and symptoms can worsen after delivery. If the disease is in remission 6 months before conception and the woman's kidneys are not involved, the chances of having a healthy baby are considered good.

SLE is treated with drugs called corticosteroids. There is no evidence that these drugs are harmful to the fetus. Your doctor may also prescribe aspirin and aspirin-like drugs to control joint pain. Usually the dosage is kept as low as possible during pregnancy to avoid effects such as fetal bleeding.

Rheumatoid Arthritis

Rheumatoid arthritis is thought of as a disease of the joints because it most often causes inflammation, pain, tenderness, heat, and swelling, particularly of the small and medium-sized joints. It is accompanied by morning stiffness and a general feeling of fatigue and discomfort. The condition can flare up and then lessen for a time, or it can become worse and worse, damaging joints. In addition, rheumatoid arthritis can affect the blood—resulting in severe anemia—or other systems of the body.

Many women find that their rheumatoid arthritis improves during pregnancy, although some have a relapse between 6 weeks and 6 months after delivery. Rheumatoid arthritis can be treated with aspirin-like drugs and sometimes other drugs during pregnancy.

Thyroid Disease

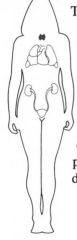

The thyroid gland can be affected by diseases that cause it to be overactive or underactive. Either can have harmful effects on the fetus. Hypothyroidism, or an underactive condition, is treated with thyroid hormone pills. Blood tests are used to determine whether the amount of hormone being taken is sufficient.

Medicines also are available to treat hyperthyroidism, or an overactive thyroid gland. The proper dose of these medicines is determined by blood tests. A patient with thyroid disease that is properly controlled during pregnancy can have a normal pregnancy.

What You Can Do

If you have a chronic disease, it is best to see your doctor before you become pregnant. If this is not possible, make an appointment as soon as you know you are pregnant. You have probably already worked out a routine for control and treatment with your family doctor or a specialist. Now your routine may need to be changed. You may have to adjust medication schedules, types, and doses to accommodate your pregnancy. If your condition is well controlled during pregnancy, your efforts will be rewarded by improving the chances of having a healthy baby.

If you are just learning now that you have some sort of illness, it can come as a shock. On top of learning about pregnancy and delivery, you must learn how to care for a medical condition. Your doctor or a specialist that your doctor recommends can help you adjust and work out a course of treatment. Pregnancy can affect medical conditions in many ways, and you may find that your condition is better after you deliver your baby.

The best actions you can take to increase the chances of having a healthy baby are to keep your condition under control, to see your doctor regularly, and to follow his or her instructions. Having a chronic medical condition that needs treatment does complicate your pregnancy, but most women with these conditions have healthy babies. You can, too.

Questions to Consider...

- Since I have a medical condition before pregnancy, should the doctor who is treating that condition be consulted?
- Is it all right to continue to take medication prescribed before I became pregnant?
- If I have high blood pressure, will it return to normal after the baby is born?
- If I have gestational diabetes, what can I do to keep it from returning later?
- How often will my condition need to be evaluated during my pregnancy?

Chapter 11

Complications of Pregnancy

Although pregnancy and childbirth are natural processes, problems can arise. The biological process is complex, and certain medical conditions can complicate pregnancy. Some complications occur when there are known risk factors. Others arise without warning. Some tend to repeat in later pregnancies, whereas others are a one-time-only event. If you have a high-risk pregnancy, it is important for your doctor and health care team to monitor your progress closely. They will adjust your prenatal care as needed and give you special attention through labor and delivery. If you suspect or detect any problems, such as the important ones described here, contact your doctor.

Vaginal Bleeding

There are many causes of vaginal bleeding in pregnancy. When bleeding occurs, the cause must be determined. To do this, your doctor may ask you for further information, examine you, or have special tests performed. Sometimes bleeding can become serious. Any bleeding should be reported to your doctor so that he or she can decide on the proper course of action based on the symptoms, signs, and stage of pregnancy. Your health and that of your fetus may depend on prompt and effective treatment.

Early Pregnancy

At the beginning of pregnancy, some women may have slight bleeding (spotting or staining). This is called implantation bleeding, and it happens when the fertilized egg first attaches itself to the lining of the uterus. Some women may confuse this bleeding with a menstrual period. When there is doubt, laboratory tests can confirm early pregnancy.

During the first 3 months of pregnancy, there is a possibility of *miscarriage*, which occurs in at least 20% of all pregnancies. Miscarriage can occur at any time during the first half of the pregnancy, but it usually occurs during the first 3 months. Sometimes when pregnancy is not progressing normally, the lining of the uterus may bleed. This is the most frequent symptom of an impending miscarriage. Another signal of a miscarriage is cramping pain, which often comes and goes, in the lower abdomen. The pain is usually stronger than menstrual cramps.

Many women who have bleeding have little or no cramping. In more than half of the women who have bleeding early in pregnancy, the bleeding stops and the pregnancy goes on to term. At other times, the bleeding and cramping become increasingly heavier and stronger, resulting in miscarriage. In some ways a miscarriage can feel like a less intense version of labor.

A woman may have repeated miscarriages. If two or three miscarriages occur in a row, the likelihood that she has an underlying problem increases. Repeated miscarriages require further studies to see whether the problem can be corrected. The woman may be advised to see another doctor with special skills to evaluate her condition.

When bleeding problems occur in early pregnancy, your doctor will most likely perform a pelvic exam and may obtain a pregnancy test. *Ultrasound* may be used to help determine whether the pregnancy is located outside the uterus (*ectopic pregnancy*) or whether miscarriage has occurred or is about to occur.

Ectopic pregnancy is a serious threat to a woman's life. It usually requires immediate major surgery to remove the fertilized egg from its abnormal position, usually from a fallopian tube. If there is doubt about whether the pregnancy is ectopic, a procedure called *laparoscopy* is sometimes performed.

If some tissue remains inside the uterus after a miscarriage, bleeding often continues. If this happens, the tissue is removed by a surgical procedure called *dilation and curettage (D&C)*. In this procedure, the cervix is widened (dilation) and tissue is gently scraped (curettage) or suctioned from the lining of the uterus.

Most miscarriages cannot be prevented. It is the body's way of dealing with a pregnancy that was not developing normally. A miscarriage doesn't mean that a woman cannot become pregnant again. Nor does it mean that anything is wrong with her health. There is no evidence that emotional stress or physical or sexual activity causes miscarriage.

Late Pregnancy

During the second half of pregnancy, any bleeding requires medical attention. The cause may be something minor such as "bloody show," the passage of a blood-tinged mucous plug from the cervix that occurs just before or at the beginning of labor. Inflammation of the cervix can also cause bleeding that is not serious.   Bleeding can be serious, however, posing a threat to the health of the woman or the fetus. All

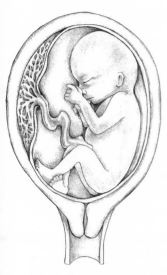

Normal pregnancy

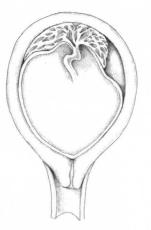

Abruptio placentae

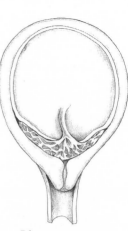

Placenta previa

bleeding in late pregnancy needs to be evaluated by your doctor. It may require admission to a hospital for more intensive care.

Heavy vaginal bleeding usually suggests a problem that involves the *placenta*. The most common causes are *abruptio placentae* and *placenta previa*. With abruptio placentae, the placenta becomes detached from the uterine wall before or during birth and vaginal bleeding usually occurs, often with constant, severe abdominal pain. The fetus may get less oxygen, which could be dangerous. With placenta previa, the placenta lies low in the uterus, partially or completely covering the cervix, the exit for the baby from the uterus. When the cervix starts to open, bleeding occurs and requires prompt care.

Contact your doctor if you have bleeding in late pregnancy. You may need to be admitted to the hospital. Ultrasound may be recommended. On occasion, a stay of several weeks in the hospital is necessary. Both abruptio placentae and placenta previa may be serious enough to require early delivery of the baby, usually by cesarean birth.

Blood Group Incompatibility

Everyone's blood is one of four major types: A, B, AB, or O. Blood types are determined by the types of *antigens* on the blood cells.

Antigens are proteins found on the surfaces of blood cells that can bring on an immune response. Type A blood has only A antigens, type B has only B antigens, type AB has both A and B antigens, and type O has neither A nor B antigens. There are other antigens, referred to as minor, that can make blood types even more specific. One of the most common of these minor antigens is the Rh factor.

As a part of your prenatal care, you will have blood tests to find out your blood type. If the mother's blood lacks the Rh antigen (Rh negative), and the father's blood contains it (Rh positive), the fetus can acquire the antigen from its father. This can result in the mother's blood being incompatible with the blood of the fetus.

Normally, during pregnancy a small amount of the fetus's blood mixes with the mother's blood. When the fetus's blood is different from the mother's blood, the mother's body may respond as if it were allergic to the fetus by making *antibodies* to the antigens in the fetus's blood. This process is called sensitization. If the antibodies the

Rh Immunoglobulin

If you are Rh negative and your partner is Rh positive, sensitization (producing antibodies against the fetus) and hemolytic disease can be prevented by injections with a blood product called Rh immunoglobulin (RhIg). It will prevent antibodies from forming, but it is not helpful if you have been sensitized and the antibodies already exist in your blood.

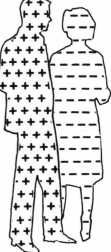

Sensitization can occur any time fetal blood mixes with the mother's blood. This could happen during pregnancy as well as after an abortion, miscarriage, ectopic pregnancy, or *amniocentesis*. RhIg will usually be given after these events to prevent sensitization and the risk of hemolytic disease in a future pregnancy. The protection from RhIg seems to last only about 12 weeks, so the treatment must be repeated at any event that could result in the mother's Rh-negative blood mixing with that of her fetus.

If a woman with Rh-negative blood has not been sensitized, her doctor may recommend that she receive RhIg near 28 weeks of pregnancy to prevent her from producing antibodies for the rest of the pregnancy. This takes care of the small number of women who can become sensitized during the last 3 months of pregnancy. If her baby has Rh-positive blood, the mother should be given another dose shortly after she gives birth. This treatment keeps the mother from developing antibodies to the Rh-positive cells from her baby that she may have been exposed to during labor and

How Rh sensitization occurs.

mother produces cross the placenta into the fetus's bloodstream, the mother's antibodies attack the fetus's blood, breaking down its red blood cells and causing anemia. This is a serious condition called erythroblastosis fetalis, also known as hemolytic or Rh disease. It can become severe enough to cause serious illness or even death in the fetus or newborn.

One of the main causes of this disease—sensitization to the Rh factor—can usually be prevented. Once antibodies are formed, they do not go away. Therefore, the best course is to prevent the mother from becoming sensitized, and thus forming antibodies, in the first place. To do this, your doctor will prescribe Rh immunoglobulin (RhIg) injections if you are unsensitized.

If you have already become sensitized, your fetus is at risk. As your pregnancy progresses, your doctor will measure the levels of antibodies in your blood. If the levels become high, special tests may be done to check your fetus's health.

delivery, removing the risk to a fetus in a subsequent pregnancy. Sensitization could occur in the next pregnancy as well, however, so repeat doses of RhIg are given with each pregnancy and birth of an Rh-positive child.

RhIg is safe for a pregnant woman. The only known side effects are soreness where the drug was injected or a slight fever. Both are temporary reactions. RhIg is prepared in a way that kills most viruses and bacteria that might have been in the blood it was made from.

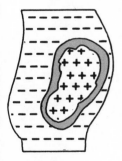
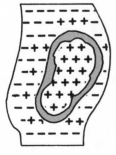
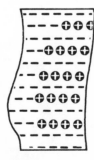
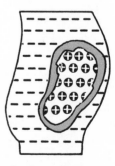

Rh-negative woman with Rh-positive fetus

Cells from Rh-positive fetus enter mother's bloodstream

Woman becomes sensitized— antibodies (+) form to fight Rh-positive blood cells

In the next Rh-positive pregnancy, antibodies attack fetal blood cells

If the fetus is anemic, it will need a blood transfusion. After 18 weeks of pregnancy, these transfusions can be given during pregnancy while the fetus is still in the uterus. If the fetus is old enough to be delivered, your doctor may decide on early delivery, and the baby can be treated in a special-care nursery.

Breech

Most babies move into the head-down position in the mother's uterus a few weeks before birth. But if this doesn't happen, the baby's buttocks, or buttocks and feet, will be in place to come out first during birth. This position is called ***breech presentation***, and it occurs in about 1 of 25 full-term births.

The causes of breech presentation are not completely clear. However, breech presentation is more common when certain other conditions are present:

- The mother has had more than one pregnancy.
- There is more than one fetus in the uterus.
- The uterus contains too much or too little ***amniotic fluid.***
- The uterus is abnormally shaped or has abnormal growths, such as ***fibroids.***
- Placenta previa has occurred.

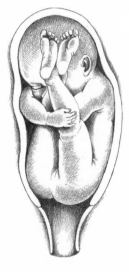
Frank breech

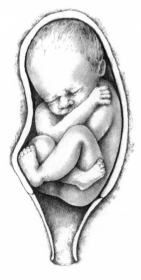
Complete breech

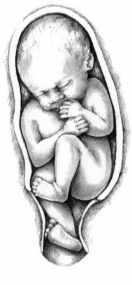
Footling breech

There are three main types of breech presentation:

1. *Frank breech*—The fetus's buttocks are directed toward the birth canal and the legs extend straight up in front of the body, with the feet near the head.
2. *Complete breech*—The buttocks are down, with the legs folded at the knees and the feet near the buttocks.
3. *Footling breech*—One or both of the fetus's feet are pointing down and will come out first.

Although most breech babies are born healthy, they do have a higher risk for certain problems than babies in the normal position. **Preterm** babies (those born 3 or more weeks early and weighing less than 5 1/2 pounds) are more likely to be breech. Birth defects are also more common in breech babies and may account for why they have not turned into the proper position before delivery. Your doctor may advise cesarean birth or may attempt vaginal delivery after carefully assessing a number of factors, such as the stage of pregnancy, the size of the baby and the mother's pelvis, and the type of breech position.

In some cases, the baby's position can be changed by a method called external version. This technique consists of manually moving or turning the baby into the head-down position. It does not involve surgery. The doctor places his or her hands at certain key points on your lower abdomen. He or she then gently pushes the baby into the head-down position, as if the baby were doing a slow-motion somersault. Often a drug is given to the mother first to relax her uterus, and the turning is done while the fetus is viewed with ultrasound.

An ultrasound exam done in advance allows the doctor to better check the condition and position of the baby, the location of the placenta, and the amount of amniotic fluid in the uterus. Before, during, and after external version, your baby's heartbeat will be checked closely. If any problems arise, efforts to turn the baby will be stopped immediately. Most attempts at external version succeed, but some babies will shift back into a breech presentation. If that happens, your doctor may try again, but external version tends to be harder to perform as the time of delivery grows closer. The best time for trying external version is several weeks before your due date.

Multiple Pregnancy

When the uterus contains more than one fetus, it is called a **multiple pregnancy.** Twins may be identical (formed from a single egg and sharing the same placenta) or fraternal (formed from two different eggs, each with its own placenta).

How Twins Are Formed

You may have wondered why sometimes twins look so much alike and other times don't seem to look the same at all. The answer has to do with how twins are formed.

Most twins are fraternal; that is, each develops from a separate egg. The ovaries usually release one egg each month to be fertilized, but occasionally two or more eggs may be released. Usually fraternal twins each have their own placenta and amniotic sac. (Sometimes these twins will be described as dizygotic, meaning two zygotes, or two fertilized eggs.) Because each twin develops from the union of a different egg and sperm, these twins look no more alike than any brother and sister do. The twins can be both boys, both girls, or one of each.

Sometimes, for unknown reasons, one fertilized egg splits early in pregnancy and develops into two or more fetuses. Two fetuses formed this way are identical (or monozygotic) twins. They share a placenta, but each usually has its own amniotic sac. Because they shared the same genetic material at the beginning, they are the same sex and usually have the same blood type, hair color, and eye color. These twins can look so much alike that even their mothers may have difficulty telling them apart.

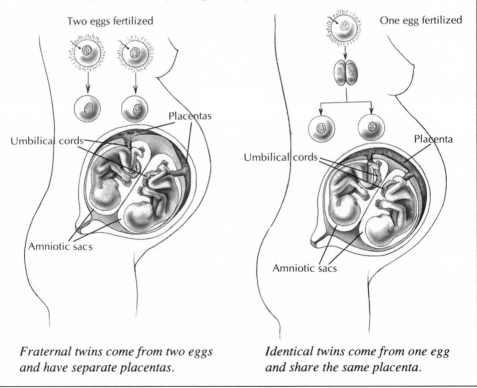

Fraternal twins come from two eggs and have separate placentas.

Identical twins come from one egg and share the same placenta.

Twins occur naturally about once in every 90 births. Triplets occur once in every 9,000 births. Black women are more likely to have multiple pregnancies than white women, whereas Oriental women are less likely. Some families are more likely than others to have fraternal twins. This is because a gene that causes the ovary to release more than one egg is passed down from mother to daughter.

Multiple pregnancies occur more often with the use of fertility drugs. These drugs are taken under close medical supervision to help ovulation occur, and they can cause more than one egg to be released from the ovaries at once.

Most multiple pregnancies are detected before delivery. Your doctor may suspect you have a multiple pregnancy if you have a family history of twins, if you gain weight more rapidly than usual, if your uterus is larger than it should be, if more than one heartbeat can be heard, or if you have taken fertility drugs. Multiple pregnancy can be confirmed by ultrasound, usually very early in pregnancy.

Multiple pregnancy increases normal discomforts of pregnancy because the uterus becomes much larger. The mother is more apt to develop high blood pressure and anemia and to have preterm labor.

If twins share the same placenta, a relatively rare complication called twin–twin transfusion syndrome can occur. In essence, one twin passes its blood to the other twin, leaving itself anemic. In its most extreme form, this syndrome can cause the twins to die.

During labor, one or both of the twins may not be in the proper position and may need to be delivered by cesarean birth. If they are both in a head-first position, it is more likely that they will be delivered vaginally. Because the uterus is so stretched out, labor may be sluggish and may not progress well. The heart rates of both twins will be monitored throughout labor, and a doctor who specializes in the care of newborns should be available when the conditions indicate.

Premature Rupture of Membranes

The cause of rupture of the membranes that hold the amniotic fluid before labor begins is not well understood. Some experts believe that when the fetus is at full term, the membranes go through changes that cause them to weaken. Other causes may be infection or bleeding. One out of every 10 women will have premature rupture of membranes (PROM) before 37 weeks of pregnancy.

When membranes rupture, the next likely event is labor. Generally, the closer you are to term, the sooner labor is likely to begin after PROM occurs. About 50% of preterm patients will be in labor within 24 hours after PROM, and more than 85% of preterm patients will be in labor within 1 week. If a woman does not go into labor, two problems can occur: the amniotic fluid and possibly the fetus could become infected, and the umbilical cord could be compressed because the fluid is not there to protect it. In general, if the fetus is not yet mature enough to survive outside the uterus, every effort is made to keep the pregnancy going. After that time, delivery is usually the best way to avoid the complications of infection.

The correct diagnosis of PROM depends on a combination of history, physical examination, and laboratory tests. Your doctor can confirm PROM by finding a pool of amniotic fluid in the vagina. A number of other tests and procedures, including ultrasound and sometimes amniocentesis, can be done when the diagnosis is not obvious. Although some of the fluid is lost when the membranes rupture, the fetus continues to produce more fluid, which may continue to leak from the uterus.

If you are found to have PROM, you may need to be hospitalized. Careful observation of mother and fetus—including frequent clinical examinations, fetal monitoring, and prompt response to changes—usually makes in-hospital care preferable.

Postterm Pregnancy

Most women (80%) give birth between 37–42 weeks of pregnancy. These pregnancies are called full term. Only 5% of babies actually arrive on the exact due date. Up to 10% of normal pregnancies extend beyond 42 weeks. These are called *postterm pregnancies*.

Knowing the gestational age of the fetus is the most important factor in diagnosing postterm pregnancy. It can be difficult, though, to precisely pinpoint the age of the fetus. Inaccurate menstrual histories, irregular menstrual cycles, and other reasons may make it difficult to predict the exact due date in every case. For this reason, doctors often use more than one method to cross-check the gestational age of the fetus (see "When Is the Baby Due?," Chapter 5). The due date should be set as early in pregnancy as possible, because it becomes less reliable when it is established later in pregnancy.

If pregnancy extends beyond 42 weeks, there could be increased risks to the health of the fetus. These risks occur in only a small number of postterm pregnancies. More than 90% of babies born between 42–44 weeks are completely unaffected by the prolonged pregnancy.

As pregnancy continues past 42 weeks, a fetus has an increased risk of:

- Abnormal heart rate—a sign that the fetus may be having problems before delivery
- *Macrosomia*—a condition in which the fetus weighs over 8 pounds, 13 ounces (4,000 grams), which can pose problems for delivery
- *Meconium* aspiration—inhalation of meconium (a greenish waste substance that is emptied from the fetus's bowels into the amniotic fluid)

It is important to identify those few fetuses at risk so that appropriate action can be taken. As a fetus passes full term, the normal functioning of the placenta may begin to decline and limit the oxygen and nutrients the fetus receives. This may result in the fetus not growing as rapidly. It may also produce less urine, thus reducing the volume of amniotic fluid in the sac. Decreased amounts of amniotic fluid may cause the umbilical cord to become pinched as a result of movements of the fetus or contractions of the mother's uterus.

There are several tests that can help the doctor check on the well-being of the fetus and the environment inside the uterus. Generally, tests are begun between 41–42 weeks of pregnancy. Some of the tests can be done by you, some are done in the doctor's office, and others are done in the hospital. Tests that may be used include *electronic fetal monitoring*, ultrasound, and amniocentesis (see "Special Tests," Chapter 5, and "Genetic Tests," Chapter 6).

If the fetus appears to be active and healthy and the amniotic fluid volume appears normal, mother and fetus may continue to be monitored at regular intervals until labor begins on its own. If the fetus appears to be at risk, delivery may be required, either by inducing labor (with the drug *oxytocin*, which causes uterine contractions) or by cesarean birth.

Why doesn't the doctor simply bring on labor at 42 weeks? First, there is often a problem in determining the exact due date. Often neither the mother nor her doctor can be certain that the fetus is fully mature and ready to be born. Second, in some women, even at this point in pregnancy, the cervix is not ready for labor to occur. Inducing labor under these circumstances makes the labor more difficult.

Women with postterm pregnancies are carefully monitored during labor. If problems occur, the baby may be delivered by cesarean birth. Once born, a postterm baby may need special care.

Preterm Labor

Preterm labor is labor that begins before the end of the 36th week of pregnancy. Normally labor begins after 37 weeks, when regular contractions of the uterus occur, along with the thinning out (efface-ment) and opening up (dilation) of the cervix so the baby can move from the uterus into the birth canal.

It is not known why some women go into labor early. Women lacking prenatal care seem to be at increased risk for preterm labor. A number of other factors have also been linked to preterm labor:

• Past pregnancies
  —Preterm labor or history of preterm birth
  —Several induced abortions
• Current pregnancy
  —Multiple pregnancy
  —Abnormalities of the uterus, such as incompetent cervix, malfor mations, or fibroids
  —Abdominal surgery
  —Infection in the mother
  —Bleeding in the second *trimester* of pregnancy
  —Underweight mother (weight less than 100 pounds)
  —Placenta previa
  —Premature rupture of membranes
  —High blood pressure
  —Maternal chronic illness

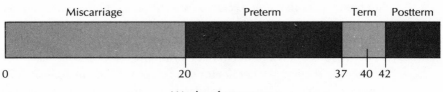

Miscarriage   Preterm   Term   Postterm

0   20   37   40 42

Weeks of pregnancy

Most women give birth between 37–42 weeks of pregnancy (term). Babies born between 20–37 weeks are preterm; those born after 42 weeks are postterm.

Signs of Preterm Labor

Sometimes the signs that preterm labor may be starting are fairly easy to detect. For example, if the membranes rupture, you may feel a continuous trickle or gush of fluid from the vagina. Other times, the signs are mild and may be harder to detect. Call your doctor right away if you notice any of these signs:

* Vaginal discharge
    —Change in type (watery, mucous, or bloody)
    —Increase in amount
* Pelvic or lower abdominal pressure
* Low, dull backache
* Abdominal cramps, with or without diarrhea
* Regular contractions or uterine tightening

If you notice signs of preterm labor, your doctor may want to see you right away. To find out whether you are actually in preterm labor, he or she will examine you to see whether your cervix has begun to change. Fetal monitoring tests are usually used to record the heartbeat of the fetus and contractions of the mother's uterus. Ultrasound may be used to estimate the size and age of the fetus and to determine its position in the uterus. You may be examined again to see whether your cervix continues to change, which is the only way to confirm preterm labor.

Preventing Preterm Birth

If labor is detected at its earliest stages and there are no signs that you and the fetus are in danger from infection, bleeding, or other complications, your doctor may try different ways to stop labor to allow the fetus more time to grow and mature:

* Bed rest
* Hydration—extra fluids given by mouth or intravenously
* Drugs that can stop or suppress uterine contractions

If you are not actually in preterm labor or if labor is stopped, you may be able to go home. At home, your doctor may ask that you feel the surface of your abdomen regularly for tightening. If you feel these contractions, count them. If you have more than six in an hour, contact your doctor. You may be in preterm labor. Some women may need to stay in the hospital for a while. This will depend on what the doctor's exam reveals and other factors.

Your Preterm Baby

Sometimes preterm labor may be too advanced to be stopped. Or there may be reasons—such as infection, bleeding, or signs that the fetus may be having problems—that the baby is better off being born right away, even if it is early. Preterm labor and delivery involve risks that require care in a hospital with special facilities. To receive this care, you may have to be moved to another hospital. Preterm babies are more likely than term babies to be delivered by cesarean birth and to have respiratory problems shortly after birth (see "Babies at Risk," Chapter 14).

Some preterm infants are kept in an incubator, which maintains proper levels of temperature and humidity.

Grieving

The death of a baby—whether before or after birth—is a profound tragedy. If you have lost a baby at any stage of pregnancy or during or after delivery, you are going through an emotionally painful time. Not only is this kind of loss usually sudden, but to many parents it also seems so unfair that the baby they have been hoping and waiting for should be taken from them.

The loss of your baby will require time for you to grieve. It is important to know that you are not alone. Ask your doctor to direct you to the support systems that are available in your community: childbirth educators, self-help groups, or clergy. You will learn that others suffering the same loss share your pain.

The grief you feel over the loss of your baby is a natural process of healing. The impact of this loss may be as great as the impact of the death of a spouse, parent, sibling, or older child. The memory will always be with you and should not be downplayed or denied.

Grief is a normal and necessary response to the loss of your baby. The grieving process that follows the death of a loved one may last from 6 months to 2 years or more.

Grieving may be described in stages, which may overlap or repeat. There is no correct way to grieve. Each family member goes through the grieving process in his or her own way:

- Shock and numbness are the mind's ways of protecting itself when first faced with a great loss. Your first reactions to the news of your baby's death may be denial, a complete lack of feeling, or an inability to grasp what death means.

- Searching and yearning begin when the initial shock phase has begun to pass. You begin to look for a reason for your baby's death. You may feel guilty or think that you did something to cause it. You may feel angry at your partner, the doctor, or a mother who has a healthy baby.

- Depression and loneliness are a part of the next phase, during which the most intense emotions begin to ease. You may feel tired and run down, sad, disoriented, and helpless. Somehow you slowly begin to get back on your feet and accept your loss.

- Acceptance is the final stage of grieving. You begin to have renewed energy, and the baby's death no longer dominates your thoughts. You find yourself resuming activities and social contacts, laughing with friends, and making plans for the future.

As you grieve, you may have other feelings or physical symptoms that are also natural and normal. These include aches and pains in the breast and arms, a tight feeling in the chest and throat, heart flutters, headaches, trouble sleeping, nightmares, loss of appetite, tiredness and fatigue, loss of memory, inability to concentrate, and fantasies about and preoccupation with images of the baby. If at any time you have concerns about what you are feeling, either emotionally or physically, don't hesitate to talk with your doctor about them. During this difficult time you need to take special care of yourself, take time to share your feelings with loved ones, and allow yourself time to heal, both physically and emotionally.

Questions to Consider...

- Is my pregnancy considered "high risk"?
- Do I have any warning signs that require action?
- Should I receive RhIg?

- My baby is in a breech position. Can it be born naturally?
- If I am carrying twins, will I probably have to have a cesarean delivery?
- Am I in preterm labor?
- Do I have premature rupture of the membranes?

Chapter 12

Infections During Pregnancy

An infection occurs when a microorganism invades a cell of the body and causes it to change. This triggers a response from the immune system, the body's form of protection that directs cells to attack the invader. The result can be symptoms of the infection, such as redness, pain, heat, and swelling, and the development of ***antibodies***, special protein molecules formed in the blood to combat a specific infection. You will not be aware of these antibodies, but you can be tested for them to see whether you have been exposed to a disease. Once you have made antibodies, you are immune to getting the disease in the future.

Infections can range from a mild cold or flu-like illness to a serious, life-threatening disease. Although a cold or flu is usually not serious to the mother or fetus, you should not treat them yourself with over-the-counter medications. Instead, consult your doctor if you have symptoms.

You can be vaccinated against some infections, but certain types of vaccines are not safe during pregnancy. A vaccine contains a small amount of either the same organism that causes the infection or an organism that is similar to the infecting agent. The amount is just enough to cause antibodies to form and make you immune but not enough to make you ill.

The best protection against infections is to avoid being exposed to them before and during pregnancy. If you think you have been exposed to an infection, inform your doctor right away. Sometimes steps can be taken to avoid serious problems and lower the risk to your baby.

Childhood Diseases

Certain infections are thought of as childhood diseases, but they can also occur in adults. Some of them can cause serious problems in pregnant women. If you've had these diseases as a child, you won't get them again. You are immune because you have developed antibodies that protect you against them. If you haven't had these diseases, it is a good idea to be vaccinated against them before your next pregnancy. Because many children aren't getting vaccinated, these diseases are becoming more widespread, making it more important to be vaccinated. If you are exposed to them during this pregnancy, your doctor may be able to treat you or your fetus to prevent the fetus from becoming ill.

Vaccines

Vaccines help prevent diseases caused by infection. Like all medicines, vaccines should be used during pregnancy only when it is necessary and safe. Ideally, a woman should have had all her vaccinations before pregnancy; but if a vaccination is necessary during pregnancy, waiting until the fourth month is generally good advice.

Some vaccines can be given safely. If you have not already been vaccinated, you may receive the following vaccines during pregnancy:

- Diphtheria
- Tetanus

Some vaccines are usually not given to pregnant women, but are safe to be used if you are likely to come in contact with the infections:

- Hepatitis B
- Pneumonia caused by *Pneumococcus*

There are other vaccines safe for pregnant women. They are not routinely given, however, unless you are likely to come in contact with the disease:
- Rabies
- Influenza
- Polio

Certain vaccines should not be used during pregnancy because they contain a live virus, which might harm the baby you are carrying:

- Measles
- Rubella
- Mumps

Exposure to measles, rubella, and mumps should be avoided during pregnancy. Women should be vaccinated against these diseases at least 3 months before they become pregnant. If you are already pregnant but not vaccinated, you should get vaccinated right after you have your baby. Vaccination is safe for you and your baby while you are breast-feeding.

Chickenpox

Chickenpox is caused by varicella–zoster virus. Adults who get chickenpox usually have more severe illness than children do. Pregnant women who get this infection are more likely than other adults to have it complicated with other illnesses, such as pneumonia.

Depending on when the infection occurs in pregnancy, it can harm the fetus in various ways. Early in pregnancy it can cause the fetus to form abnormally or even die. When the mother gets chickenpox before a week from delivery, the baby may be born with chickenpox or may be protected by the mother's antibodies. Babies born with chickenpox usually recover completely. If the mother gets chickenpox within a week of delivery, however, there is no time for her antibodies to develop and cross the *placenta* to protect the baby. These babies are more likely to become seriously ill and may die.

Because it is so easily transmitted, pregnant women who are not immune to chickenpox should stay away from infected persons, especially near the time of their delivery. They should also avoid contact with a person who has shingles, because this disease is another form of infection with varicella–zoster virus. If a pregnant woman does become infected, a drug called varicella–zoster immunoglobulin may prevent her from developing serious illness if it is given within 96 hours of exposure. Varicella–zoster immunoglobulin may not protect the fetus from the infection, however. Infants whose mothers were infected a few days before birth should receive varicella–zoster immunoglobulin after birth to prevent them from developing serious illness, too. A vaccine for the virus that causes chickenpox is being developed.

Fifth Disease

Fifth disease is so called because it was the fifth to be discovered among a group of diseases that cause fever and skin rash in children. It is caused by human parvovirus B19. A common childhood disease, fifth disease usually results in a mild flu-like illness. About half of all adults have antibodies to fifth disease, showing they have been exposed to it.

Infection with parvovirus B19 is cause for concern during pregnancy. Women who have long-term, close exposure to the disease, such as mothers who have an infected child at home or teachers in a school with an epidemic, are at higher risk of becoming infected than women with more casual exposure. If you are exposed to fifth disease in the first *trimester* or early second trimester, you are at increased risk of *miscarriage*. Still, the miscarriage rate is only about 1–2% higher than normal. When infection occurs later in pregnancy, it can cause anemia in the fetus and may require treatment.

If you may have been exposed to fifth disease during pregnancy, talk to your doctor. He or she may be able to test you for signs of the virus.

Rubella (German Measles)

There are different types of measles caused by various viruses. Most do not cause problems during pregnancy. The type that has the most severe effects during pregnancy is caused by rubella virus and is known as German measles. Since 1969, when a vaccine for rubella became available, preschool and young school-age children have been vaccinated. It has been estimated that about 75–80% of the population is protected against rubella by the time they reach childbearing age because they have been exposed to the disease, have had it, or have been vaccinated. Once infected with rubella virus, you are immune for life, even if the infection doesn't actually make you ill.

It is fortunate that so few people are now susceptible to rubella, because the virus can cause birth defects and long-term disorders in babies who are exposed to the virus while their mothers were pregnant. The risk depends on when infection occurred during the fetus's growth and development. If infection occurred during the first month, about 50% of the babies will be affected. By the third month, the risk is lowered to about 10%. The most common problems include cataracts (an eye problem that can cause blindness), heart defects, and deafness—together called congenital rubella syndrome. Other disorders, such as diabetes, can develop later in life.

As a routine part of prenatal care, each pregnant woman is tested for antibodies to show whether she is immune to rubella. If there are signs that a woman is not immune but may have been exposed to rubella or if she develops symptoms (fever, rash, swollen lymph glands), she will be tested again. If the diagnosis of rubella infection during pregnancy is confirmed, a type of immunoglobulin may be given. If the woman has been exposed to rubella but has not developed the disease, the immunoglobulin may prevent her from becoming ill. It will not prevent the fetus from being affected, however.

Because rubella can have such a severe impact on the fetus and because nothing can be done during pregnancy to protect the fetus, it is best that a woman receive the rubella vaccine before she becomes pregnant. A woman who has not had rubella or the vaccine could be vaccinated just after delivery, before she becomes pregnant again. Although the vaccine does not cause congenital rubella syndrome, the virus in the vaccine may be able to infect the fetus. Therefore, it is best to wait 3 months after receiving the vaccine before trying to become pregnant. Should you receive the vaccine during early pregnancy, however, the risk that the baby will have a problem is very low.

Mumps

Less than 10% of all cases of mumps, a disease caused by a virus, occur in people older than 15 years. Mumps is less contagious than measles or chickenpox. This means that mumps is uncommon during pregnancy. If you do get mumps during pregnancy, your symptoms are likely to be no worse than if you were infected before pregnancy. When a woman develops mumps in the first trimester of pregnancy, however, it doubles her chance of having a miscarriage. Mumps may also cause **preterm** labor. Because this infection is so rare during pregnancy, it is not clear whether it is linked to birth defects.

The vaccine against mumps that is given to children has greatly limited the number of pregnant women who are exposed to the disease. Having mumps as a child also gives you protection. Many people who don't remember having had mumps might have had a very mild case that would still provide protection. If you are one of the few women who is susceptible to getting mumps, it may be a good idea for you to be vaccinated after you give birth. Because there is a very small chance that the vaccine could hurt your fetus if you were vaccinated during pregnancy, it is not given to pregnant women.

Cytomegalovirus

Cytomegalovirus (CMV) infection is hard to detect because those who have it often do not have symptoms. When symptoms occur, they are similar to those of mononucleosis: fever, tiredness, swollen lymph glands, and sore throat. Rarely does CMV produce serious illness in an adult. Even though about 60–70% of the general population have signs of previous infection, about 90% of those previously infected have never been ill.

CMV infection poses a problem during pregnancy and the postpartum period, when it can be passed to the baby through the placenta, the vagina, or breast milk. Unlike other viral infections, CMV can still recur in a woman who has previously been infected and developed antibodies. The risk of the fetus becoming infected is greatest during the first (primary) bout of infection in the mother. Although the overall risk of primary infection in pregnant women is low (about 2%), the chance of the fetus becoming infected at the time of the mother's primary infection is fairly high. Recent studies have shown that among mothers infected with CMV during pregnancy for the first time, about 50% of the fetuses are infected with CMV in the uterus. Only 10% of these fetuses showed signs of disease, however. Those infants who do have symptoms at birth are at higher risk for severe illness, death, or handicaps. Some of the problems that can arise as a result of CMV infection are *jaundice*, microcephaly (having a very small head and often being mentally retarded), deafness, and eye problems.

There is no treatment for CMV infection, and because it so rarely causes symptoms when a pregnant woman is infected, screening or general testing is not effective. It is not known exactly how CMV is spread, but it can be passed from close person-to-person contact through saliva, urine, or sexual contact. The best protection is to avoid contact with infected persons and to use good personal hygiene, especially hand-washing.

Hepatitis

Hepatitis is a viral infection that affects the liver. Two forms of hepatitis are commonly identified: type A and type B. Hepatitis B is the most serious during pregnancy and can be transmitted by blood, kissing, or sexual contact.

Hepatitis B virus (HBV) can cause chronic infection. Even though there may be no outward signs of the disease, the person infected can become a carrier and develop long-term problems such as cirrhosis, or hardening, of the liver and possibly liver cancer. The rate of chronic HBV infection in the general population is low. It tends to be much higher in certain populations:

• Women of Asian, Pacific island, or Alaskan Eskimo descent
• Women born in Haiti or sub-Saharan Africa
• Women with a history of:
  —Work in a health care field
  —Liver disease
  —Work or treatment in a hemodialysis unit
  —Work or living in a home for the mentally retarded
  —Rejection as a blood donor
  —Multiple blood transfusions
  —Household contact with an HBV carrier or person receiving hemodialysis

—Multiple sex partners

—Illicit intravenous drug use

About 80% of infants born to women with chronic HBV infection become infected, usually during delivery. Of these infants, most will also become chronic carriers of the virus and be at risk for the long-term consequences of HBV infection.

During pregnancy, HBV infection should be diagnosed as early as possible so that hepatitis B immunoglobulin can be given to reduce the severity of the illness. Unfortunately, it may be difficult to diagnose hepatitis in pregnancy because its symptoms are nausea and vomiting, which often occur in the natural course of pregnancy. The diagnosis can be confirmed by testing for hepatitis virus ***antigens*** or antibodies in the blood. It is recommended that all women be tested routinely for HBV early in pregnancy. Women in high-risk groups should be vaccinated to avoid becoming infected.

If a woman develops HBV infection during pregnancy, she will be treated with bed rest, diet, and liquids. Arrangements will be made for the baby to receive HBV vaccine and hepatitis B immunoglobulin immediately after birth to guard against the risk of infection and long-term problems.

Lyme Disease

Lyme disease is caused by a bite from an infected tick. When the tick bites, it injects bacteria into the body that cause disease. The first sign of Lyme disease is a sore that often looks like a bull's-eye. This sore may go away, but the infection remains. It spreads to the joints, causing arthritis, and can cause muscle pain. ***Antibiotics*** such as penicillin or tetracycline will usually cure the infection. If untreated, it can progress to attack the heart and nervous system.

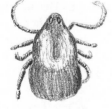

Wood tick (top) and deer tick (bottom).

There have been reports that the bacteria the tick carries can pass from an infected mother to the fetus through the placenta. The result might be birth defects or miscarriage. However, it is too soon to tell for sure whether these problems are caused by Lyme disease or by something else. Ticks can carry diseases other than Lyme disease.

It is wise for pregnant women to avoid heavily wooded areas and to wear long-sleeved shirts and long pants in areas where ticks can be found.

Sexually Transmitted Diseases

Sexually transmitted diseases are the most common infectious diseases in the United States except for colds and flu. Although some can be cured, others cannot. All sexually transmitted diseases can lead to serious complications, and some are especially harmful during pregnancy. The sexually transmitted diseases for which testing is available, and their effects, are described in Chapter 1.

Toxoplasmosis

The parasite that causes toxoplasmosis lives in some mammals, such as cats. Humans can become infected by eating raw or undercooked meat, especially lamb or mutton, or by coming into contact with cat feces. Toxoplasmosis causes only mild illness in adults, and often those exposed have no symptoms. About 20–40% of the general public has been exposed to toxoplasmosis.

Toxoplasmosis creates a problem in pregnancy only when the mother is first infected at that time. When the infection first occurs in pregnancy, the fetus is also infected in about one-third of the cases. Of these, another one-third will have signs of the disease. The risk of infection is highest in the last 3 months of pregnancy, but the infection is most severe when it occurs in the first 3 months. Because the risk to the fetus occurs only when a woman becomes ill during pregnancy, routine blood testing of pregnant women is not recommended.

The mother often does not show signs of infection. When they occur, she may notice swelling of the lymph glands in the cervical area. Other symptoms include fever, fatigue, sore throat, and rash. Infection during pregnancy can cause the baby to be born prematurely or to be too small. It can also cause fever, jaundice, eye problems, or other long-term problems.

A combination of antibiotics is used to treat toxoplasmosis, but these drugs are not safe to use during pregnancy because of their toxic effects. Infected babies are treated soon after birth, and early treatment can prevent long-term problems.

The best way to protect against toxoplasmosis is to avoid being exposed to it. Be sure meat is thoroughly cooked. Cats should be fed only store-bought cat food and be kept from eating mice, which could harbor the parasite. If your cat goes outside often, it is a good idea not to hold it close to your face. Keep the cat off of your bed blankets, pillows, and sheets. Because cat feces are not infectious during the first 24 hours, cat litter should be changed daily, preferably by someone else. Once feces do become infectious, they stay that way for a long time. Pregnant women should wear rubber gloves or avoid gardening in areas where there are cat feces. Always wash your hands well, with soap and water, after touching soil, cats, or uncooked meat or vegetables.

Urinary Tract Infections

Urinary tract infections are common in pregnancy. Severe infections can cause problems for both mother and fetus. Some urinary tract infections can be detected only by tests—there may be no symptoms to let you know that you have an infection. Your doctor will be testing you regularly, however, to avoid any problems. Some symptoms linked with a urinary tract infection, such as painful urination, can be caused by other problems, such as infection of the vagina or vulva. To help your doctor make the correct diagnosis, you should bring any changes to his or her attention.

Cystitis is a lower-tract (bladder) infection. Its symptoms include an increased need to urinate, burning and pain during urination with possible signs of blood in the urine, and discomfort in the lower abdomen. With proper treatment, this condition usually clears up right away.

Pyelonephritis is an upper-tract (kidney) infection. Its symptoms are similar to those of cystitis. However, pyelonephritis can also cause chills, fever, rapid heart rate, and nausea or vomiting. This condition can cause premature labor or septic shock. If you have pyelonephritis, you will probably be hospitalized for treatment and careful monitoring. Under these conditions, most patients recover within 48 hours.

Questions to Consider...

- If I can't remember being vaccinated or having certain diseases, what should I do if I am exposed to one of them?
- If I have another child who is sick, what can I do to keep from getting sick too?
- If I get a cold, will it hurt the baby? Can I take cold remedies?
- Which vaccinations have I received? When?
- Do I work with people who are at risk of hepatitis?
- How can I tell if I have urinary tract infection?
- If I own a cat, what precautions should I take with removal of the litter?

Labor, Delivery, and Postpartum

Section III

Labor, Delivery, and Postpartum

For the past several months, you have been seeing your doctor regularly and learning how you are changing and how your baby is growing. As you near the end of your pregnancy, you are probably waiting eagerly for your baby to be born. You may be a little nervous about what is to come—most women are. One of the best ways to relax and enjoy this special experience is to know what is happening to you and what to expect. Learning as much as you can will help make your baby's arrival a pleasant, exciting time.

After delivery and your return home, your life will change. Your new baby will demand care and attention 24 hours a day. Attention to your needs, as well as the support from others close to you, can make meeting this challenge a little easier.

Chapter 13

Labor and Delivery

Awaiting the birth of a child is an exciting and anxious time. Most women give birth between 37–42 weeks of pregnancy. However, there is no way to know exactly when you'll go into labor. Labor that begins as much as 3 weeks before or 2 weeks after your due date still is considered normal.

As you plan for the birth, you can take steps to help your delivery go more smoothly. These steps should be discussed with your doctor before the time comes. The following are some questions that should be answered in advance:

- When should you call your doctor?
- How should you reach your doctor after office hours?
- Should you go directly to the hospital or call the doctor's office first?
- Are there any special instructions your doctor wants you to follow when you think you are in labor?

There are also quite a few things to think about before it is time to make the decision to go to the hospital. You may not have time to think about them once labor begins. They include some of the following:

- *Distance.* How far do you live from the hospital?
- *Transportation.* Is someone available to take you at any hour of the day or night, or do you have to call and find someone?
- *Time of day.* Depending on where you live, it may take longer to get to the hospital during rush hours than at other times of the day or night.
- *Time of year.* Bad weather or other factors may make the trip longer.
- *Home arrangements.* Do you have other children who must be taken to a babysitter's home, or must other special arrangements be made?
- *A suitcase for the hospital.* It is often a good idea to pack two suitcases—a small overnight case with just a few personal items, such as a toothbrush and a comb, to take with you, and a larger suitcase with all of your other things to be brought later. Do not bring jewelry or large sums of money to the hospital.

Packing Your Suitcase

It's a good idea to find out in advance what items the hospital provides for you during labor and what you will need to bring yourself. Talking with hospital staff and other women who have delivered there can help you to plan. A childbirth educator is also a good source of information. Here are some items you may wish to consider:

- Comfortable gown and robe
- Slippers
- Several pairs of socks
- Hair brush
- Toothbrush and toothpaste
- Glasses (contact lenses will be removed during labor)
- Lip balm
- Tennis balls (for counter-pressure)
- Talcum powder or cornstarch
- Ties or barrettes for long hair
- Watch
- Pad and pencil
- Change for vending machine and phone
- Phone numbers of people whom you plan to call after the birth
- Clothes for both you and the baby to go home in

It may be a good idea to rehearse going to the hospital to get a sense of how long it could take. You may wish to plan an alternate route to the hospital in case you run into a delay on the preferred route.

How Labor Begins

It is not certain exactly what causes labor to begin. Most women can tell when they are in labor. However, in about 10% of the cases, it may be difficult for a doctor or woman to know, and a period of several hours of observation is necessary.

Labor begins when the cervix begins to open, or dilate. The uterus, which is a muscle, contracts at regular intervals, causing the abdomen to become hard. Between contractions, the uterus relaxes, causing the abdomen to soften. Certain changes take place that may signal the approach of labor.

True Versus False Labor

You may experience periods of "false" labor in the form of irregular contractions. These irregular contractions, called ***Braxton–Hicks contractions,*** may become quite uncomfortable. They usually occur more often in the afternoon or evening, after physical activity, or when you are tired.

False labor can occur just at the time when labor is expected to start. Thus, it is sometimes difficult to tell false labor from true labor, and you may be fooled. Don't be upset or embarrassed if you react by thinking labor is beginning. Sometimes the difference can only be

How Labor Begins

Sign	What It Is	When It Happens
Feeling as if the baby has dropped lower	*Lightening.* This is commonly referred to as the baby "dropping." The baby's head has settled deep into your pelvis.	From a few weeks to a few hours before labor begins, especially with first babies
Discharging a thick plug of mucus or an increase in vaginal discharge (clear, pink, or slightly bloody)	*Show.* A thick plug of mucus has accumulated at the cervix during pregnancy. When the cervix begins to open wider, the plug is pushed into the vagina.	Several days before labor begins or at the onset of labor
Discharging a continuous trickle or a gush of watery fluid from your vagina	*Rupture of Membranes.* The fluid-filled sac that surrounded the baby during pregnancy breaks (your "water breaks").	From several hours before labor begins to anytime during labor
Feeling a regular pattern of tightening or what may feel like a bad backache or menstrual cramps	*Contractions.* Your uterus is a muscle that tightens and relaxes. The hardness you feel is from your uterus contracting. These contractions may cause pain as the cervix opens and the baby moves through the birth canal.	Usually at the onset of labor

determined by a vaginal exam to detect changes in your cervix that signal the onset of labor.

There are ways to distinguish between true and false labor. One good way is to time the contractions. Time how long it is from the start of one contraction to the start of the next one. Keep a record for an hour. During true labor:

- The contractions last about 30–70 seconds.
- They occur at regular intervals (usually 5 minutes or less).
- They don't go away when you move around.

Keep in mind that timing of labor pains is hard to do accurately if the contractions are slight. It's best to be cautious—don't wait too long to call your doctor if you think you are going into labor, especially if it isn't your first labor.

There are other signs that should prompt you to call your doctor and to think about going to the hospital:

- Your membranes rupture (your "water breaks"), even if you are not having any contractions.
- You are bleeding from the vagina (but not if it is just "show").
- You have constant, severe pain with no relief between contractions.

You can be ready for labor when it occurs by knowing what to look for and what to expect. By being prepared, with your questions answered in advance, you can focus your attention on the birth of your baby when the time comes.

True Versus False Labor

Type of Change	False Labor	Labor
Timing of contractions	Often are irregular and do not consistently get closer together (called Braxton–Hicks contractions)	Come at regular intervals and, as time goes on, get closer together
Change with movement	Contractions may stop when you walk or rest, or may even stop with a change of position	Contractions continue, despite movement
Location of contractions	Often felt in the abdomen	Usually felt in the back coming around to the front
Strength of contractions	Usually weak and do not get much stronger	Increase in strength steadily

The Language of Labor

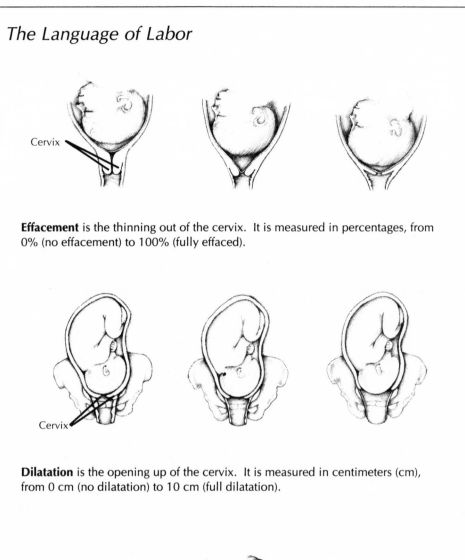

Cervix

Effacement is the thinning out of the cervix. It is measured in percentages, from 0% (no effacement) to 100% (fully effaced).

Cervix

Dilatation is the opening up of the cervix. It is measured in centimeters (cm), from 0 cm (no dilatation) to 10 cm (full dilatation).

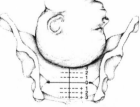

Station is the relationship of the baby's head to a bony landmark in the pelvis.

The Support Person's Role

Many fathers want to become an active partner in the birth of their child. If a father does not want to get involved in the delivery itself, there are other ways to give support. The father can be involved during childbirth preparation, during labor, and after the delivery by assuming an active role in caring for you and the baby. Caring can take many forms, and you can decide with the father what is best in this family-centered approach to childbirth.

The support person need not be the father, though; any close relative or loved one can help a woman as she prepares for birth. During delivery, the partner may stand near the head of the delivery bed, beside the mother's shoulder. From this position, the partner can offer emotional and physical support while seeing the birth of your

Stages of Labor

On the average, the entire labor process lasts about 12–14 hours for a first birth and usually shorter for subsequent births. The labor process is divided into three stages. During each stage, certain changes take place in your body and in the way you feel. Every woman is different and every labor is different. You will not experience each labor the same way.

First Stage

The first stage begins when the cervix starts to open and ends when your cervix is completely opened (fully dilated). The onset of regular contractions may be a sign that labor is beginning, but a woman can have contractions and not be in labor. The first stage is usually the longest, and it occurs in three phases: early (latent), active, and transition.

Early Phase
- The cervix dilates to 4–5 cm.
- Mild contractions begin at 15–20 minutes apart and last 60–90 seconds.
- Contractions gradually become more regular, until they are less than 5 minutes apart.

- A small amount of "show" may occur during this stage.

Active Phase
- The cervix dilates from 4 to 8 cm.
- Contractions become stronger and progress to 3 minutes apart, lasting about 45 seconds.

Transition Phase
- The cervix dilates from 8 to 10 cm.
- Contractions occur 2–3 minutes apart and last about 60 seconds.

child just as you do. The partner may also prefer to stand at the end of the bed, next to the doctor, or even take pictures to record the event.

If a problem arises, your support person may be asked by the doctor to leave the delivery room. The doctor may not be able to take time to explain the reasons for this request at the moment. In the best interest of the mother and baby, partners should leave right away. Further explanation will be given when time permits.

Admission

Once it appears that you are in labor, you will be admitted to the hospital obstetric unit. There your doctor, the nurses, and other members of the health care team will work together in caring for you before, during, and after your delivery.

Besides helping your cervix to efface (thin out) and dilate fully, the contractions during labor are helping the baby to come through the birth canal. Throughout labor, the baby is moving deeper into the pelvis and farther down the birth canal. The baby's head and body move and turn for the easiest fit possible through the pelvis. The contractions continue to help the baby to be born, usually head first.

Second Stage

When your cervix is fully dilated, the first stage ends and the second stage begins. This stage continues until the birth of the baby. It may last up to 2 hours or longer, especially during a first labor.

- Contractions may slow to 2–5 minutes apart during the second stage of labor and last 60–90 seconds.
- Pushing with your contractions begins at this stage.

Third Stage

This last stage begins after the baby is born and ends when the *placenta* is expelled. It is the shortest stage and may last from just a few minutes to 15–20 minutes.

- Contractions are closer together and may become less painful in the third stage of labor.
- The placenta separates from the uterine wall and is delivered.

Once you have been admitted and the status of your labor has been assessed, you will be prepared for delivery. The steps in preparation vary, but generally you can expect the following:

- You'll be asked to remove all your clothes and to put on a special gown.
- You'll be examined to determine how far labor has progressed.
- Some of the hair in the vaginal area may be shaved.
- You may be given an enema to empty your bowels.

A needle may be placed into a vein in your arm or wrist when you are in active labor. This needle is attached to a tube that will supply your body with fluids, medications, or, during an emergency, blood. This assembly is called an intravenous (IV) line.

Your doctor may not be with you the entire time while you are in labor, but he or she will be available to check on your progress. A team of nurses will care for you throughout the process. They will note your vital signs, such as heart rate and blood pressure, as well as the timing of the contractions to monitor the progress of labor. The baby's heartbeat will be checked by the nursing staff on a regular basis during labor. Labor and delivery nurses are trained to help you through the physical and emotional demands of labor. In teaching hospitals, resident doctors are often part of the team. Your labor may be in the same room used for delivery, or you may be moved to a delivery room for the actual birth.

You will be asked to sign a consent form when you enter the hospital and possibly again if cesarean delivery is to be done. These documents vary somewhat, but most spell out the procedure, who will be the responsible surgeon, what condition it is intended to remedy, and the risks. Your signature verifies your understanding of these factors and gives permission for your doctor to provide care. Read this form carefully, and be sure to ask questions about anything you don't understand.

Monitoring

Fetal heart rate monitoring is used to check on the condition of a fetus in the mother's uterus during labor. Certain changes in the heart rate of the fetus can signal a problem, so every woman receives some form of close monitoring while she is in labor. Better knowledge about what can happen to the fetus during labor, along with improvements in equipment, has allowed more accurate analysis of the results of fetal monitoring. Fetal monitoring cannot prevent a problem from occurring, but it can help your doctor be alert to warning signs.

There are two methods of fetal monitoring: ***auscultation*** and ***electronic fetal monitoring***. The method used depends on the equipment and nursing staff available and whether there are any complications.

Auscultation

Listening to the fetal heartbeat at certain intervals is called auscultation. The timing is based on how far along the mother is in labor and whether any risk factors are present. The heartbeat can be heard by one of two ways:

1. A stethoscope (a device through which a heartbeat can be heard) is placed on the doctor's or the nurse's head, with the open end pressed on the mother's abdomen. The device amplifies the heartbeat of the fetus, allowing the doctor or nurse to hear it through ear pieces.

In auscultation, a special stethoscope is used to listen to the fetal heartbeat.

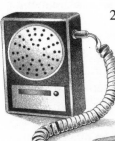

2. Doppler ***ultrasound*** uses sound waves to create an audible signal of the fetal heartbeat. A small, hand-held device is pressed against the mother's stomach. It emits sound waves that are reflected back from the fetus as signals of the heartbeat that anyone in close range can hear (see "Special Tests," Chapter 5, for more information about ultrasound).

Doppler ultrasound uses a small, hand-held device.

When auscultation is used, the heart rate of the fetus is usually monitored and recorded after a contraction. The doctor or nurse will place his or her hands on the mother's stomach to feel contractions of her uterus. The mother is not confined while the doctor or nurse is not listening to the heart. She can move about as she pleases as long as her doctor believes that there are no medical reasons that would indicate bed rest. There are no known risks with auscultation.

Electronic Fetal Monitoring

The second type of monitoring electronically measures the fetus's heart rate on an ongoing basis. The electronic equipment provides a continual record of information that can be read by the doctor or nurse. There are two methods of electronic fetal monitoring:

1. *External monitoring* requires that two belts be placed around the mother's abdomen to hold two small instruments in place. One instrument computes the fetal heart rate by means of ultrasound. The other instrument measures the length of uterine contractions and the time between them.

2. *Internal monitoring* can be used only after the fetal membrane (the amniotic sac in which the fetus grows in the mother's uterus) is broken. A small device called an electrode is attached to the scalp of the fetus to record the fetal heart rate. Sometimes a thin tube called a catheter may be placed in the uterus to measure the strength of uterine contractions. Most women who have had these procedures done during labor report feeling only minor discomfort, about the same as a routine examination of the cervix.

Sometimes a combination of internal and external devices is used. The internal scalp electrode records the fetal heart patterns, and the external pressure monitor records uterine contractions.

With internal fetal monitoring, an electrode is attached to the scalp of the fetus to record the fetal heart rate.

With either internal or external monitoring, information about the mother and the fetus is relayed to a small machine. This information is recorded on a long strip of paper, producing a tracing that is read by your doctor or nurse. The tracing shows patterns of the fetal heart rate in relation to uterine contractions.

Both internal and external methods have advantages. The external fetal monitor does not require the cervix to be dilated or the membrane around the fetus to be broken. Internal monitoring, though, may give more accurate information about the fetus's condition and the strength of the mother's uterine contractions. Neither method affects the progress of labor.

When the monitoring equipment is in use, the mother may be asked to stay in bed, because that makes it easier to keep the monitor in place. Most women readily adapt to the monitor and are often reassured by the sounds of the fetal heartbeat.

When risk factors are present, a woman is more likely to receive electronic fetal monitoring. Although complications from electronic fetal monitoring are extremely rare, infection or slight injury may arise where the electrode is placed on the baby's head.

Electronic fetal monitoring is just one of many ways your doctor may assist you with your delivery. A number of factors are involved in deciding to use it. You should discuss any questions you may have about it with your doctor as you prepare for the delivery of your baby.

Pain Relief

Many women take childbirth preparation classes to learn what to expect during labor and delivery. They also learn breathing methods, relaxation techniques, and other ways of coping with pain and discomfort during childbirth. These classes can be quite valuable, and some women are able to use these techniques to get through childbirth without needing pain medication. Other women find that using these techniques combined with some medications relieves the discomfort of labor and birth. Throughout delivery, your nurse will be available to reassure you and help make you more comfortable.

Your wishes will be taken into account in deciding what type of pain relief is best for you. Many other factors, including your well-being and that of your baby, will affect this choice. Often your doctor will not be able to tell you exactly what kind of pain relief you will receive until you are in labor or are ready to deliver. Many times these choices must be left open and flexible until your doctor sees how your labor is going. Also, you may not always be able to have medication just when you feel you need it.

Pain-relieving medications fall into two general categories. *Analgesia* is the relief of pain without total loss of sensation. A person receiving an analgesic medication remains conscious. Although analgesics don't always completely stop pain, they do lessen it. *Anesthesia* refers to the total loss of sensation. Some forms of anesthesia cause a loss of consciousness, whereas others remove the sensation of pain from specific areas of the body while the patient remains conscious.

The decision to use a pain medication and what type to use will depend on several factors. Not all types of pain medications are available at all institutions, and not all doctors are able to give every type. Often the choice cannot be made until labor is under way. Your doctor may work with an anesthesiologist—a doctor who specializes

Easing Discomforts

In addition to the breathing and relaxation techniques you can learn in child-birth preparation classes, there are other ways of relieving discomfort you may feel during labor. Massages often feel good. You may want your partner to rub or firmly press on your lower back. You might also want to have an ice pack bottle for your back. Frequent position changes can make you more comfortable. During contractions, you or your partner can try rhythmic stroking of your abdomen. Rubbing a little lotion on your skin first will reduce pulling on your skin. If you have leg cramps, massage or change of position can help relieve them.

You should not eat or drink during active labor. To keep your mouth moist, however, you may be allowed to suck on ice chips.

It is best to try to remain relaxed, especially between contractions. In early labor, when contractions are farther apart, watching television, playing games, or listening to music may be soothing. It may be helpful to try to rest or sleep during this time to prepare for the later, more active phases of labor, when more energy is required. When contractions are closer together and stronger, rest in between and take slow, deep breaths. If you become warm or perspire, cool, moist cloths may be soothing. Feeling warm is usually just a sign that you are working hard.

in pain relief—in selecting the best method for you, depending on how your labor or delivery is going and the state of your health. And, of course, the effect of the medication on your baby must also be considered.

Systemic Analgesia

Systemic analgesics are often given in the form of an injection into a muscle or vein. They lessen the intensity of pain without causing loss of consciousness. They act on the whole nervous system, rather than on one particular area. Sometimes other drugs are given with systemic analgesics to relieve tension or nausea.

Like other types of drugs, pain medications can have some side effects. Most are minor, such as drowsiness and decreased ability to concentrate. Also, because these drugs can slow the baby's reflexes and breathing at birth, they are given in small doses and are usually avoided shortly before delivery.

Serious side effects are uncommon. In addition, doctors and other health care professionals know how to administer these drugs in ways that will reduce the chances of side effects.

Pudendal Block

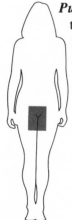

Pudendal block is given shortly before delivery as an injection to block pain in the perineum. It is especially helpful for numbing the perineum before an episiotomy is performed. It also relieves the pain you may have around the vagina and rectum as the baby descends through the birth canal. Pudendal block is considered one of the safest forms of anesthesia, and serious side effects are rare.

Paracervical Block

With **paracervical block**, a local anesthetic is injected into the tissues around the cervix. It relieves the pain as the cervix dilates to allow the baby's head to descend into the birth canal. It also helps relieve pain from contractions of the uterus. Although paracervical block provides

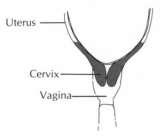

good pain relief, it wears off quickly. Sometimes it causes slowing of the baby's heart rate. This effect is usually temporary, but in rare cases it persists and the doctor may decide to deliver the baby quickly. Because of the effects on the fetus, this form of anesthetic is not used as often as it once was. When it is used, the heart rate of the fetus is closely monitored.

Epidural Block

Epidural block, another form of local anesthesia, affects a larger area than any of the other methods described. It causes some loss of feeling in the lower half of the body; the extent of numbness will depend on the drug and dose used. An epidural block is injected into the lower back. Medication is placed into a small space (the epidural space) outside the spinal cord compartment, where the nerves that receive sensations from the lower body pass to reach the spinal cord. This kind of anesthesia is helpful for easing the pain of uterine contractions, the pain in the vagina and rectum as the baby descends, and the pain of an episiotomy. In stronger doses, epidural blocks can also be used to block pain during cesarean birth.

You will be asked to sit or lie on your side with your back curved outward and to hold this position until the procedure is completed. The procedure itself should cause little discomfort. Your back will be washed with an antiseptic, and a tiny area of the skin will be numbed with a local anesthetic. After the epidural needle is in place, a small tube (catheter) is usually inserted through it, and the needle is then withdrawn. That way, small doses can be given through the tube at a later time or the medication can be given continuously without your having to have another injection. Low doses are used because they are less likely to cause side effects in the mother and baby and result in less numbness of the legs. It may take a short while for the drug to take effect. Although you will be much more comfortable, you may still be aware of your contractions. In some hospitals, a woman can be given medication through the tube following the delivery to help relieve her pain for as long as 24 hours after birth.

With modern techniques that use low doses of medication, most women can deliver normally with an epidural anesthetic. If the mother is very numb, however, it may be harder for her to bear down and help the baby move through the birth canal. In this case, it may be necessary for the baby to be delivered with *forceps* or ***vacuum extraction***, special instruments that are placed around or attached to the baby's head to help guide it out of the birth canal.

Epidural block can have some side effects. It may cause the mother's blood pressure to drop, which in turn may slow the baby's heartbeat. Preventive steps are taken to avoid this problem: before the mother receives the medication, fluids are given through an intravenous line (IV) in her arm, and she is positioned on her side to help circulation.

Serious complications are rare. If the covering of the spinal cord is punctured during the procedure, the patient may get a severe headache, which untreated can last for a few days. This headache can often be treated with a fairly simple procedure. If the drug enters the spinal fluid, the muscles in the patient's chest may be temporarily affected, making it hard to breathe. If the drug enters a vein, it could cause dizziness or, rarely, seizures. Complications from epidural anesthesia are very unusual, however. Special precautions are taken by the highly qualified doctors who perform it to decrease the likelihood that problems will occur.

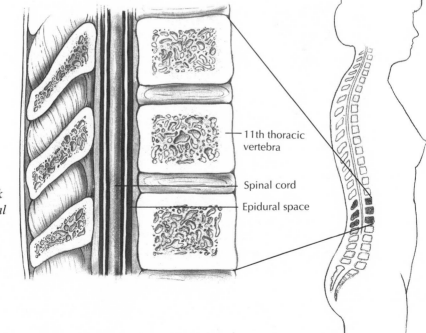

Insertion points for spinal block and epidural block anesthesia.

11th thoracic vertebra

Spinal cord

Epidural space

Spinal Block

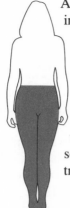

A *spinal block*, like an epidural block, is given as an injection in the lower back. A small amount of medication is injected into the spinal fluid and numbs the lower half of the body. It provides good relief from pain and starts working quickly, but it lasts only an hour or two. Spinal block is usually given only once during labor, so it is best suited for pain relief during delivery, particularly if forceps or vacuum extraction is needed. It is most often used for cesarean birth. Spinal block can sometimes cause some of the same side effects as epidural block, which are treated in a similar way.

General Anesthesia

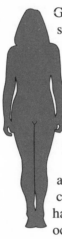

General anesthetics are medications that produce loss of consciousness. The mother will not be awake or feel any pain during delivery. General anesthesia is not used to relieve the pain of labor. It is used for cesarean birth and, occasionally, emergency vaginal delivery.

A rare but serious complication of general anesthesia occurs when food or acid from the stomach enters the windpipe and lungs and causes injury. Because of this, you should not eat solid food once labor has started.

Whether you should have general, spinal, or epidural anesthesia for a cesarean delivery will depend on your condition and that of the baby, as well as the reason you are having it. When there is an emergency or when bleeding occurs, general anesthesia often is preferred.

Local Anesthesia

Just as your dentist uses a drug to numb areas in your mouth, your doctor can use a local anesthetic to ease pain during delivery. Local anesthetics usually affect a small area and so are especially useful when the doctor has to do an *episiotomy*—a small cut, or incision, in the *perineum* (the area between the vagina and rectum)—before the baby is born. Local anesthetics are also helpful during the repair of this incision or of any tears that might have occurred during birth.

One advantage of local anesthesia is that it rarely affects the baby. After the anesthetic wears off, there are usually no lingering effects. The main limitation of these drugs is that they do not relieve the pain of contractions during labor.

Helping Labor Along

Sometimes a doctor may choose to induce, or start, labor. Labor is induced when the risks of delivery for the mother or fetus, or both, are less than the risk of continuing the pregnancy. The same methods used to induce labor can also speed up labor that is not progressing well. Conditions under which a doctor may choose this procedure include, but are not limited to:

• Rupture of membranes not followed by labor
• Postterm pregnancy
• Pregnancy-induced hypertension
• Maternal medical problems such as diabetes and lung disorders
• *Chorioamnionitis* (inflammation of the membrane surrounding the fetus

Before the doctor decides to induce labor, he or she will do various tests to find out whether it can be done safely. The fetus's condition will be checked. If it will be born preterm, the doctor will check the *lecithin/sphingomyelin (L/S) ratio*. Lecithin and sphingomyelin are substances found in the *amniotic fluid*. When there is twice as much lecithin as sphingomyelin, the fetus's lungs should be mature enough to allow it to survive outside the uterus. The cervix will also be examined to see if it is thin and dilating for labor. If your doctor decides labor should be induced, fetal monitoring will be done at the same time to monitor the well-being of the fetus.

There are several ways to induce labor, one of which is breaking the membranes. This is done during a vaginal exam and is usually no more painful than a regular exam. Most women go into labor within 12 hours after their membranes rupture. Breaking the membranes also allows the doctor to perform internal electronic fetal monitoring, if necessary.

You may also receive a drug called *oxytocin* to help bring on contractions or to make them stronger. If your doctor decides that oxytocin is the best way of inducing labor, you will first have an IV started. The oxytocin is given by a pump that accurately measures how much of the drug you receive.

As with any drug, there are some risks with oxytocin. Your fetus may not respond well to contractions produced by oxytocin. If fetal monitoring shows that your fetus may be having problems, you may be given oxygen to breathe and IV fluids and may be positioned on your side, and the oxytocin infusion may be slowed or stopped.

Delivery

When your cervix is fully opened, the baby begins to move down the birth canal, usually head first. You will feel an urge to push, or bear down, or have a bowel movement. Tell your doctor or nurse when you begin to feel this way.

Generally, you should try not to bear down with each contraction in early labor, and you should try to relax between contractions. After the cervix dilates completely, you will be told when to push and when to avoid pushing by controlling your breathing as the baby moves down the birth canal. Your doctor watches the baby's progress and will tell you how to help it along. Your doctor may perform an episiotomy to prevent tears in the perineum. The baby's head will be born first. Then the baby's body rotates so that first one shoulder and then the other appears. The baby's body follows quickly.

Episiotomy

During delivery, when your baby's head crowns—appears at the opening of the vagina—the tissue of the vagina becomes very thinly and tightly stretched. Sometimes, even if the tissue is stretched as much as possible, it is difficult for the baby's head to fit through without tearing the mother's skin and perineal muscles. To prevent your muscles from tearing and to relieve some of the pressure on your baby's head, your doctor may make a small cut in the vagina and perineum while the area is numbed with a local anesthetic. This procedure is called an episiotomy. This is one of the most common operations in the United States: 50–90% of first-time mothers and 25–30% of mothers who previously had a child will have an episiotomy when their child is born.

Just after birth, your baby is held with the head lowered to help keep the amniotic fluid, mucus, and blood from getting into its lungs. A small bulb syringe may be used to suction the mouth and nose. The baby is then dried and is warmed with blankets, heat lamps, or a heated bassinet. Drops or ointment to prevent infection will be put into the baby's eyes, and identification bands will be placed on you and the baby before you leave the delivery room. The baby's hand and foot prints may also be taken.

After the birth, you and your baby are still attached by the *umbilical cord*. Your doctor will cut the cord and deliver the *placenta*. Your uterus will be massaged to keep it firm and hard. Your doctor will examine your vagina, cervix, and perineum. If you had an episiotomy, your doctor will repair it at this time, as well as any tears that may have occurred.

To assess the health of your newborn, your doctor will use a method called the *Apgar score*. This method, described in Chapter 14, is used to identify babies that may need extra attention.

Unless you or your baby is having medical problems or complications, you will probably be able to hold the baby. If you had decided to breast-feed, you may be able to start at this time. It is an especially rewarding feeling for you and your partner to be close to your baby just after birth.

Forceps and Vacuum Extraction

Sometimes it is necessary for the doctor to help delivery along by using forceps or vacuum extraction. These techniques are used when the fetal heartbeat slows or becomes irregular, when the baby's position makes delivery difficult, or when the mother is too tired to push. You will be given an anesthetic before forceps or vacuum extraction is used.

A forceps is a surgical instrument that looks like two large spoons. The doctor inserts the forceps into the birth canal, places them around the baby's head, and gently delivers the baby.

Delivery may be assisted with forceps (above) or a vacuum instrument (right).

Delivery

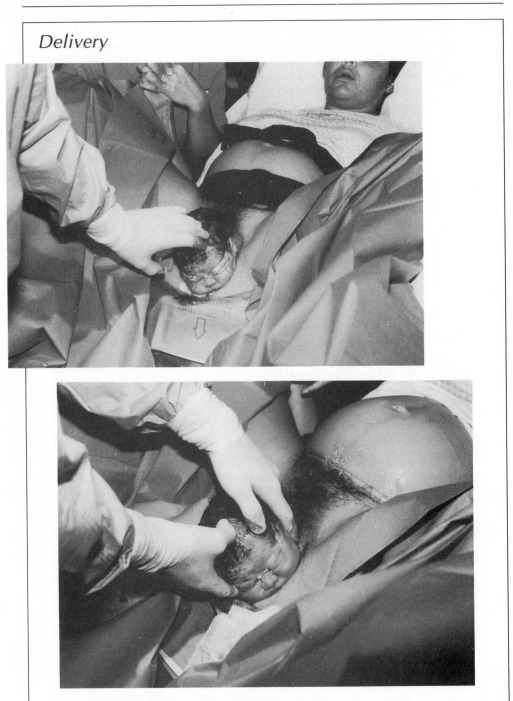

As the baby's head emerges (above), *the doctor helps guide it out of the birth canal* (below). *The baby's body follows quickly.*

The Birth of a Baby

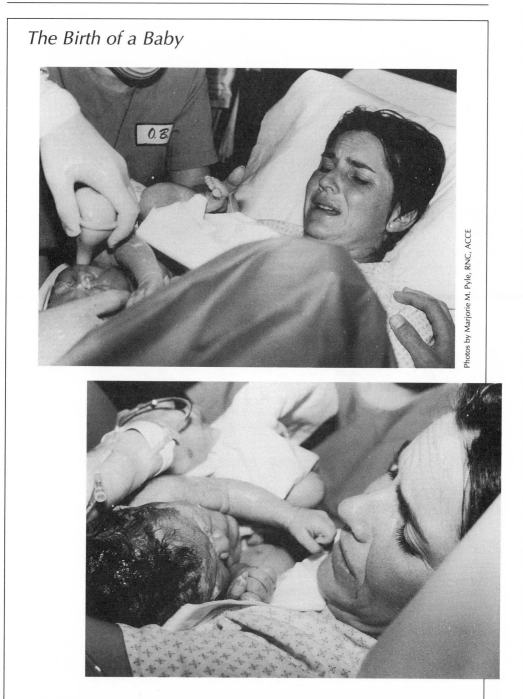

Photos by Marjorie M. Pyle, RNC, ACCE

Immediately after delivery, the baby's airway is suctioned (above) *before the baby is held by the mother* (below).

Vacuum extraction is similar to forceps delivery, but in this technique a plastic cup is attached to the baby's head by using a vacuum pump, and the baby is gently pulled from the birth canal.

Cesarean Birth

If for some reason it is not safe for the baby to be delivered through the vagina, cesarean birth may be needed. A cesarean birth may be planned for reasons known in advance, or it may be needed because of problems that arise unexpectedly. A cesarean delivery should not be viewed as a failure on the part of either the mother or the doctor, nor should it detract from the fulfillment of the childbirth experience. The method of delivery is always less important than the overall goal: a healthy mother and baby.

There are many reasons why a cesarean birth might be chosen as the safest way to deliver a baby:

- *Cephalopelvic disproportion*, or CPD, in which the baby is too large to pass safely through the mother's pelvis
- Fetal stress, a warning that the baby is having difficulty during labor and may need to be delivered right away. One of the reasons this could occur is that the cord is compressed.
- Placental problems that could occur with vaginal bleeding
- *Breech presentation,* in which a baby is born buttocks or feet first or in other unusual positions

When it is not safe for the baby to be delivered through the vagina, a cesarean delivery will be performed.

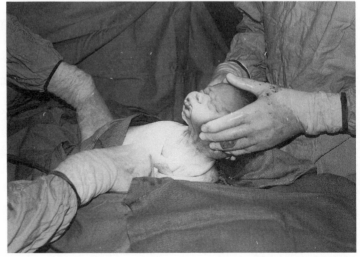

Photo by Marjorie M. Pyle, RNC, ACCE

There are many other reasons for cesarean birth. Medical illness such as diabetes or high blood pressure may require delivery at a time when vaginal delivery cannot be safely performed.

Before a cesarean birth is performed, the nurse prepares you for the operation. The lower part of the abdomen is washed and may be shaved. The bladder is next to the area where the cesarean birth is performed. To lower the risk of injury to the bladder, it is drained of its urine by a catheter placed in the bladder before surgery to keep it empty. An IV will be inserted in a vein in your hand or arm, permitting fluids to be given intravenously during the operation. Any medication that you might require may also be given through the IV. After you are taken to the operating room, anesthesia is administered. If general anesthesia is chosen, you will be unconscious during the delivery. If spinal or epidural anesthesia is used, you will be awake but numb from just around the nipples down to your toes. The anesthesiologist will discuss the various types of anesthesia available (described earlier in this chapter) and will consider your wishes.

In many hospitals, the patient's partner or another support person may stay with the woman in the operating room for the cesarean birth. This could depend on whether the mother is awake, the urgency of the operation, and local hospital policy. If the support person is present at the birth, he or she will change into appropriate clothing provided by the hospital before entering the operating room.

A cesarean birth involves the following steps:

1. The doctor makes an incision through the wall of the abdomen. It may be a vertical incision from the navel to the pubic bone, or it may be a transverse incision that extends from side to side, just above the pubic hairline.
2. An incision is next made in the wall of the uterus, through which the baby is delivered. This incision may also be either vertical or transverse. The transverse incision is made in the thinner, lower part of the uterus and is the preferred incision if the situation permits. It is preferred because there is less blood loss and it heals with a stronger scar. However, a vertical incision of the uterus is sometimes needed for other reasons, such as certain positions of the baby or *placenta previa.*
3. After the delivery of the baby and placenta, the incisions are closed with sutures and clips.

Because cesarean birth is a surgical procedure, it can involve certain risks:

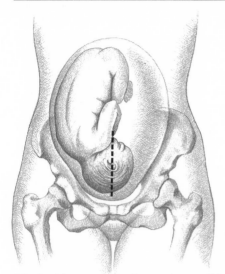

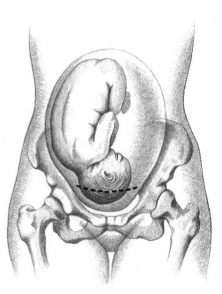

The incision made in the uterine wall for cesarean birth may be vertical (left) *or transverse* (right). *The type of incision made in the skin may not be the same as the type of incision made in the uterus.*

- Infection of the uterus and nearby pelvic organs
- Increased blood loss, sometimes severe enough to require a blood transfusion
- Blood clots in the legs, pelvic organs, and sometimes the lungs
- Decreased bowel function
- Longer recovery time and hospital stay

   Many maternity centers provide childbirth classes, programs, or support groups designed just for couples who may need cesarean delivery. If you have questions or concerns about cesarean birth, you should bring them to the attention of your doctor so that they may be answered before the birth of your child.

Vaginal Birth After Cesarean Delivery

At one time it was thought that once a woman had a cesarean birth, she would always have a cesarean birth in any subsequent pregnancies. Today, though, most women who have had cesarean births are being encouraged to attempt to give birth through the vagina, if no risk factors are present. In fact, most of these women have successful vaginal deliveries.

There are several reasons to consider a vaginal birth after a previous cesarean delivery:

- *Less Risk.* A vaginal delivery has fewer complications for the mother than cesarean birth. A cesarean birth requires major surgery and is performed with anesthesia. As with any operation, there is risk of infection, bleeding, and transfusion (getting blood), as well as problems that can occur with any surgery and anesthesia. With a vaginal birth, there is no abdominal incision, so these risks are much lower.

- *Shorter Recovery.* The mother's stay in the hospital is likely to be shorter after a vaginal delivery, and she will have less discomfort than after a cesarean. The average time spent in the hospital is usually a few days longer after a cesarean birth than after a vaginal birth. Recovery at home is usually faster after vaginal birth, too. Women who deliver by cesarean birth may need to limit their activity for a few weeks to allow the incision time to heal. Those who deliver vaginally can resume normal activities sooner.

- *More Involvement.* Some women wish to be awake and fully involved in the birth process. Sometimes general anesthesia is used during a cesarean delivery, in which case the mother is not awake and cannot experience the actual birth. There also may be more limits on the presence of others in the delivery room during a cesarean birth.

In addition to your own wishes, there are a number of medical factors that will be weighed in the decision about how your baby will be born. One of these is the type of uterine incision that was used in your previous cesarean. Your doctor will need to consult your medical records from the previous cesarean birth to verify which type of uterine incision was used. This is because the main risk to both you and your baby during an attempted vaginal birth is separation or rupture of the scar left by that incision. Rupture may be more or less likely, depending on what type of incision was used.

There are three types of uterine incisions used for cesarean delivery:

- The transverse incision, which is made across the lower, thinner part of the uterus, is usually preferred for cesarean delivery. It heals with a stronger scar and is least likely to result in complications in a subsequent vaginal delivery.
- The low vertical incision is an up-and-down cut made in the lower, thinner area of the uterus. The risks involved in vaginal birth after this type of uterine incision are not well defined. If you have had this type of incision, discuss the options with your doctor.

- The classical (high vertical) incision is an up-and-down cut made in the upper part of the uterus. This was once the most common type of incision used in cesarean births. Unfortunately, a complete rupture, or opening, of the scar is more likely to occur during labor if a classical incision was used in a previous cesarean delivery. This can result in serious bleeding that can pose danger to both the fetus and the mother.

It is important to realize that, in a cesarean delivery, the type of incision made in the skin may not be the same as the type of incision made in the uterus. For this reason, it is not be possible to tell what type of uterine incision you had just by looking at the scar on your abdomen. If it is not possible to determine this, your doctor will help you decide whether you may be a good candidate for vaginal birth. Although you may plan for a vaginal delivery, keep in mind that something could arise that would require a cesarean delivery.

After all the medical factors have been weighed and your own wishes have been considered, you may prefer to attempt vaginal delivery. Because an attempt to deliver vaginally after a previous cesarean birth carries some risk, certain safety measures will be taken during labor and delivery. It is important that the setting in which you give birth be equipped to perform an emergency cesarean delivery.

During labor, electronic fetal monitoring may be used to detect unusual changes in the fetus's heart rate. If a problem does occur during labor, you may need to have an emergency cesarean delivery.

For most women, the benefits of attempting vaginal birth after a previous cesarean delivery outweigh the risks. Even women who have had two or more cesareans can safely attempt to give birth through the vagina. With careful monitoring, proper support, and no major medical problems, most women who attempt vaginal birth after a previous cesarean delivery do so safely and satisfactorily.

After Delivery

You will be observed closely after delivery to be sure that there are no problems. Your blood pressure, pulse, and temperature will be taken, your uterus will be massaged, and you will be examined for signs of heavy vaginal bleeding or infection. After a period of staying in bed, you are encouraged to move about with help. A nurse or other adult should stay with you during your first several times out of bed.

If you have had a cesarean birth, you will usually stay in bed for 6–8 hours. Some hospitals are encouraging early contact between patient and baby after a cesarean birth. In these hospitals, if the baby's condition at birth permits, the parents and child stay together in the operating room and the recovery area.

Soon after surgery, the catheter is removed from the bladder. You should then be able to resume urinating without difficulty. Occasionally the catheter has to be reinserted. Fluids will be given intravenously until you are able to eat and drink. For most women, intravenous fluids are given for 1 or 2 days.

During the first several days after a cesarean birth, the abdominal incision is uncomfortable. Medication for pain relief can be given.

After delivery, most hospitals provide for mother, father, and baby to spend some time together. A perfect time to begin learning about your baby is while you are still in the hospital. Examining your baby from head to toe and noticing special characteristics is a joy for every mother. Sometimes, however, the baby does not look or act as you think a baby should. Most of the time, nothing is wrong—you are just noticing normal characteristics of a newborn. Many mothers have formed images of older babies while they are pregnant and are surprised at what a newborn really looks like. Take advantage of the availability of your doctor and nurses to answer your questions and to reassure you. Nurses who work in maternity units specialize in teaching new parents infant-care skills.

Children who visit their mothers after the birth of a sibling have been reported to respond better to their mothers and new brother or

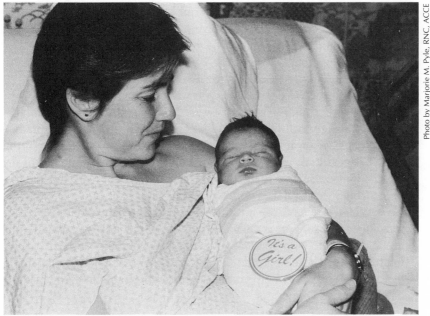

Photo by Marjorie M. Pyle, RNC, ACCE

sister than children who do not. Most hospitals have policies for sibling visitation:

- Children should not have been exposed to known communicable diseases such as chickenpox.
- Children should not have fever or symptoms of acute illness such as upper respiratory infection.
- Children should be prepared in advance for their visit.
- Parents should ensure that children are supervised by a responsible adult during the entire hospital visit.

Be sure to find out before your delivery what your hospital's policies are with regard to sibling visitation. You may often choose to restrict visits to allow more time for you to rest and get to know your baby.

Discharge

If you have had a normal vaginal delivery, you will be discharged from the hospital in about 2 days, depending on your particular circumstances. If your baby has had complications in the delivery, he or she may need to stay longer.

The length of the hospital stay after a cesarean birth depends on the reason for the cesarean birth and on the amount of time you need to resume normal functions. In most cases, a woman leaves the hospital 3–5 days after a cesarean birth.

Other procedures may be done in the hospital before discharge, possibly lengthening the stay. The mother may decide to have post-partum sterilization. If the baby is a boy, the parents may decide to have him circumcised (see Chapter 14).

Before you are discharged, you will be given instructions to follow in case a complication or emergency occurs. You should make arrangements for follow-up examinations of yourself and your infant. Your doctor will want to examine you about 4–6 weeks after the birth. Your baby will probably be examined by a doctor once a month for the first 3 months. Be sure to have your infant safety seat ready for the trip home from the hospital. Use it every time your baby is in the car.

When you leave the hospital to care for the baby at home, remember that support is available, either individually or in small group classes, to help you learn some of the beginning skills of motherhood. These will often include feeding, bathing, and diapering the baby, all of which help you feel more comfortable in the way you handle your newborn.

Questions to Consider...

- When should I call the doctor once labor begins?
- Am I prepared to go to the hospital at any time?
- Can I review in advance any forms I may be asked to sign?
- What type of fetal monitoring will I have?
- What forms of pain relief will be available?
- When is my follow-up visit?
- What special instructions will I need at the time of discharge?

Chapter 14

The Newborn Baby

The first sight or sound of your baby will make a lasting impression. What you are seeing and hearing is not a beginning, but an adjustment. Your baby is moving from one environment—within the mother's uterus—to another, outside. After being surrounded by fluid and mother, the baby must adjust to being surrounded by air and the wide world.

While hidden away in the uterus, the fetus goes through a remarkable process of growth involving both physical changes and development of the ability to function. Birth is but a point in this gradual process that begins with conception and continues into adulthood. At birth you can begin to watch your baby grow and develop, right at a time when major changes are occurring.

The heart and lungs in particular go through major changes during birth and adjustment to life outside the uterus. Although some risk goes along with these changes, in most births they occur without problems. Doctors and nurses are trained to care for the baby. Often all that is required is for them to follow some basic steps to ensure that everything is going well.

The physical and functional changes you will see in your baby around birth and in the early days afterward involve the baby's appearance, size, and responses. When you understand the process of growth and development that occurs as your baby adjusts to a new life, you will be more able to relax and enjoy the natural course of events while you care for your baby.

Appearance

At birth, babies can appear quite different than they do a few days or weeks later. Television and magazines often use infants who are 1–3 months old to represent newborns. As a result, many parents are surprised when their baby looks different than they expected.

A baby who has just emerged into the outside world often is covered with a greasy, whitish coating called **vernix**. There may also be traces of blood and other material. This is normal. The arms and legs may be drawn up and, while moving, tend to return to the position last assumed in the uterus. A baby's face and head may appear quite

A newborn baby (below) *looks much different from one that is 1–3 months old* (right).

Photo by Michael Dodd

different at birth than they will later. In the uterus the head was under pressure. The face is likely to appear a bit swollen and the eyes puffy. Skull bones are not fused and can be flexible; therefore, some babies have heads that appear elongated or even pointy. Babies born by cesarean birth can have the same appearance if their mothers went through labor before delivery; if labor did not occur, their faces and heads may appear more like those of babies several days old. When given their baby after birth, parents often first look at the face and then at details such as the hands and feet. Doctors and nurses do that as well, but they also listen to the heart and lungs with a stethoscope to check the baby's health. They may want to check more than once while you are getting to know your baby to make sure that organs have withstood labor and are adjusting to life outside mother's uterus.

Skin Color

In the time just after birth, skin color may not be uniform. In addition to the whitish vernix covering the skin, some newborns may have a bluish or gray appearance, especially of the hands and feet. This is usually temporary.

After a few days some babies' skin becomes yellow. This condition is called *jaundice*. This is caused by a buildup of bilirubin, a greenish yellow substance that is produced when red blood cells are broken down as a natural process of the body. The liver removes bilirubin from the body. During pregnancy, the *placenta* and mother's liver remove bilirubin from the fetus. The baby's liver cells don't begin to function to remove bilirubin until a few days after birth.

Parents should not be overly concerned about jaundice that appears a few days after birth. Although high levels of bilirubin can be toxic to the baby's nervous system, the levels in most babies are not likely to cause problems. Before the liver begins to function naturally, the amount of bilirubin in the blood can be checked and the baby can be placed under fluorescent lights, which lower bilirubin levels.

Weight and Age

Everyone wants to know how much a baby weighs at birth. The hospital will give you that figure, usually in pounds and ounces (doctors and nurses express weight in grams; for example, 2.2 pounds = 1,000 grams = 1 kilogram). There is no such thing as a proper or "good" weight, but there is a range that is considered normal. Problems can occur if a baby is too big or too small.

The normal age of a baby at birth is between 37–42 weeks from the first day of the mother's last menstrual period. Together, the

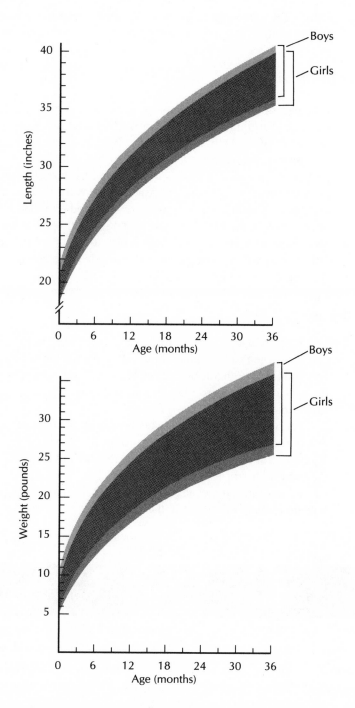

Average growth of boys (■*) and girls (*■*), from birth to 36 months, in length* (top) *and weight* (bottom).

baby's age and weight can show whether a fetus has grown normally before birth.

Response to Birth

As a part of her interest in a baby's response to birth and life on its own, Dr. Virginia Apgar developed a score to assess several key indicators of the baby's well-being. Practically all babies are assigned an *Apgar score*, taken at 1 minute after birth and again at 5 minutes, as part of the monitoring process. The five characteristics are assigned a number between 0–2, and the Apgar score is the total of those numbers. Although the Apgar score is a good tool that assists in understanding the baby's progress at a given time, it does not by itself show how well the baby did before birth or what the future will hold. Other signs will also be checked to provide more complete information on the baby's general health.

The First Cry

The lungs replace the placenta at the time of birth as the organ that carries oxygen to the blood. Not only must the lungs be able to become filled with air, but all related structures—such as muscles and the airways leading from the mouth and nose—must be ready to function.

A baby spontaneously takes breaths at the time of birth. Why this occurs is not clear. It appears to result from the baby being stimulated at birth and from changes that take place in the makeup of the baby's blood.

After birth, the change in pressure between the lungs and the air outside leads to the filling and expanding of the lungs with air. The

Apgar Score

Component	Score		
	0	**1**	**2**
Heart rate	Absent	Slow (< 100 beats/min)	>100 beats/min
Respirations	Absent	Weak; hypoventilation	Good, strong cry
Muscle tone	Limp	Some flexion	Active motion
Reflex irritability	No response	Grimace	Cough or sneeze
Color	Blue or pale	Body pink; extremities blue	Complete pink

vocal cords are developed and can move, and the baby cries. In addition to the first cry, babies will often respond to handling with cries.

Many babies will cry loudly and often at birth, but some don't cry. Some babies begin to breathe without crying. After birth, a baby can be self-supporting at the oxygen levels found in room air, both at rest and during activity. Breathing will be watched closely by birth attendants, and measures will be taken to help if a baby's breathing is not adequate.

Circulatory Changes

Blood moves to and from the placenta through vessels (two arteries and a vein) in the ***umbilical cord***. At the time of birth, the placenta comes loose from the inside of the uterus and is expelled. Thus, a major flow of blood that is involved in respiration, nutrition, and other functions of the fetus stops suddenly. At the same time, blood flow to the lungs increases dramatically.

Just after birth, when the baby's lungs are filling with air and receiving more blood, doctors and nurses often listen to the chest carefully with a stethoscope. In addition to the sound of air entering the lungs, they can often hear sounds or murmurs associated with the changes in blood flow that are a normal part of the baby's adjustment. You may also see doctors feel the pulse in locations such as the arm or groin. Parents shouldn't be alarmed when they see these examinations done; it is part of the routine assessment of the status of the baby.

Temperature Control

The healthy fetus gives off heat through the placenta to its mother, and it is protected from heat loss by the surrounding warmth of mother. At birth, the baby enters an environment that is much cooler than the mother's uterus. Being wet, the baby is at risk for serious heat loss through evaporation. Studies have shown that the temperature of most babies drops during birth. This loss can be kept to a minimum by drying and wrapping the baby just after birth.

Newborns have controls to maintain their body temperature, but these systems are not as efficient as those in older children and adults. Environments that are too hot or too cool can overwhelm the newborn. Normal infants in the first week after birth need some clothing, such as a cotton shirt or gown, in addition to a diaper and perhaps a light blanket. The room should be draft free and not too warm or too cool (70–75°F) or dry (35–60% humidity).

Nervous System

A baby's basic reflexes, such as those that control breathing, function
well. The baby is able to interact with people and respond to sound
and light. Parents may notice a complex reflex action, such as the
startle or Moro reaction, in which a newborn extends the arms, legs,
and head and then draws the arms back to the chest in response to a
strong stimulus such as a sound. Sight, hearing, and pain sensation are
present from birth but are more easily recognized as the baby matures.

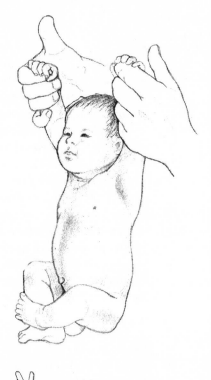

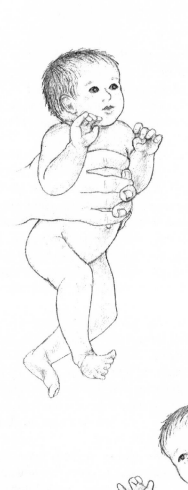

*A newborn's reflexes
include* (clockwise
from left) *stepping,
grasp, and startle
reflexes.*

Gastrointestinal System

The placenta was the main source of food for the fetus before birth. After birth, the baby is able to feed by sucking and swallowing milk through the mouth and moving it into and through the intestinal tract. Although unable to handle an adult diet, a baby can digest carbohydrates, proteins, and fat soon after birth. Feeding can take place early the first day. The fetal intestine contains a dark, tarry substance called ***meconium*** that is usually seen within 24 hours when the first bowel movement occurs.

Behavior

As newborns adjust to life outside the uterus, they have similar biologic needs and respond with a limited set of behavioral reactions. Beyond this, however, each baby expresses a unique personality. Wide variations in how each baby behaves and interacts with people are evident from birth. Some seem quiet and subdued and indeed may have seemed quiet in the womb; others show lusty crying and vigorous kicking.

After the stress and physical adjustments of birth, the baby often has a brief period (an hour or so) of being alert and may suckle if put to the mother's breast. The baby may then fall asleep or be drowsy for the next several hours or even few days.

At first, babies spend most of their time sleeping (in short intervals that total 14–18 hours per day) with only brief periods of alertness. Some babies spend more time awake from the beginning and are fussy rather than quiet and alert. Others will spend long stretches sleeping and gradually awaken to a quiet state. Parents can alter sleep/wake patterns to help babies adapt to a fixed schedule. For example, by encouraging the baby to stay awake during the day and by ignoring fussiness and avoiding anything that keeps the baby awake at night, parents may be able to alter cycles. The need to feed during the night may continue for 2–3 months after birth and sometimes longer, so some interruption at night cannot be avoided.

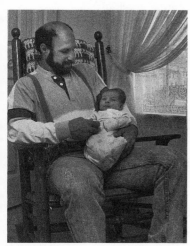

Photo by Earl Dotter

Bonding is the magic feeling that a mother has toward her infant shortly after birth. Not all mothers feel this way right away. The baby may not look as the mother expected, or a difficult birth, such as preterm delivery, may prevent bonding. In a short time, a few days at most, interaction will become closer as mother and baby adapt to each other. Attachment is the gradual process of developing a loving relationship between a baby and his or her parents over time. The difference between bonding and attachment can be compared to love at first sight versus the building of a loving relationship.

Care of the Baby

From the start, newborn babies are well equipped to function. However, they are not independent and need help in many ways.

Feeding

Breast milk, including the *colostrum* of the first 2–4 days, is designed just for infants. Breast-fed infants have fewer feeding problems, tend to be less constipated, and have fewer infections and allergies than babies who are bottle-fed. If bottle-feeding is chosen, mothers are fortunate to have modern formulas that come close to human milk.

If a mother is nursing, the first feeding can be tried as soon as the baby's condition is stable after birth. Although only a small amount of fluid may be produced at the time, the attempt is often rewarding to mothers. When the baby is being fed formula, the first feeding should take place within 6 hours of birth. A baby is born with all the reflexes necessary to nurse and will know what to do when offered the breast. When the nipple is placed in the baby's mouth, the baby will begin to suck, causing milk to flow.

Newborns will nurse about 3 minutes on each breast at each feeding for about the first 24 hours. This time gradually increases

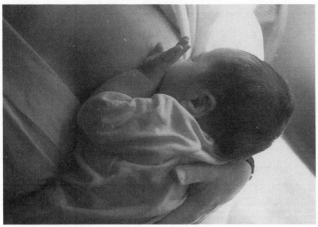

until the baby nurses for 15 minutes or longer on each breast. Although most of the milk is taken in the first 5–10 minutes, the infant may want to suck longer. It is not necessary that the baby nurse at both breasts at one feeding. Just try to remember which breast was used and offer the other at the next feeding.

Photo by Michael Dodd

Your baby may want to nurse only every 4 hours or as often as every 1/2 to 11/2 hours. Keep in mind that babies are not initially programmed to eat at regular intervals. Don't be surprised if your baby nurses for 15 minutes, falls asleep for 2 hours, and then nurses from each breast for 15 minutes. Every baby is different and will set his or her own pattern; there are no strict rules. You can tell whether your baby is getting enough milk if it wets at least six diapers every 24 hours.

Feeding provides contact between mother and baby that builds their relationship. The routine should be adjusted to allow enough time for this important activity and to make it as comfortable as possible.

Bathing

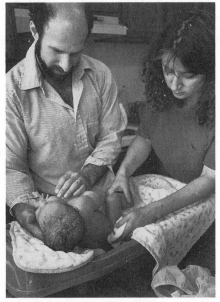

Photo by Earl Dotter

Cleanliness is important for health and appearance. It is convenient, but not absolutely necessary, for a baby to have a full bath in the first few days after birth. The baby's skin can be cared for without a total body bath. Sponge baths, especially around the diaper area and in skin creases, will do fine. Vernix does not have to be removed and may have a beneficial effect. Bland soap is helpful but not necessary.

When a bath is given, it should not take place until after the baby has made his or her adjustment after birth and has a stable temperature. Demonstrations of bathing are frequently a part of the hospital stay after birth. If discharge is planned before bathing is demonstrated and a mother feels uncertain about it, she should ask for special instruction before leaving.

Eye Care

Shortly after birth, hospital personnel place an ointment or solution in a newborn's eyes. This is done to guard against possible infection of the eye during birth. Additional treatment is not necessary unless evidence of infection, such as redness or discharge, occurs. If such signs appear, you should speak with a doctor or nurse. Otherwise, all that is necessary is gentle wiping of the closed eye with moist cotton or cloth to keep the area clean.

Cord Care

The stump of the umbilical cord will usually fall off in 7–10 days. Care of the cord area is important due to the risk of infection. The area should be kept clean and dry, but it does not need to be covered. Some doctors suggest using ointment or other substances during the first week or so. If redness spreads to the surrounding skin, call your doctor.

Diapering

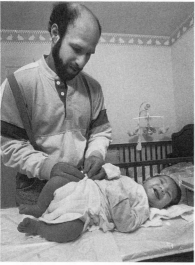

Photo by Earl Dotter

Newborns usually stool and urinate in the first 24 hours. Some will begin in the delivery room, and others will wait more than 24 hours. If this function is delayed, the doctor may want to explore the reason. Most urinate 6–18 times and stool as much as 7–8 times daily. Cloth or disposable diapers are used for cleanliness.

Dressing

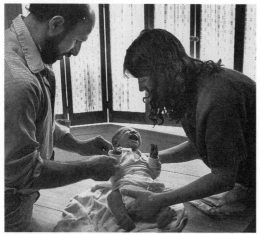

Photo by Earl Dotter

In general, babies need about the same number of layers of clothing as their parents. One-piece baby suits made with soft, nonirritating material and with easy access to the diaper area are practical. In warm weather only a diaper may be needed. In air-conditioned rooms, outside, or on cold days, infants may need more layers than adults because they don't move as much. The environment can guide your choice of clothes to bring to the hospital for the baby to wear home.

Circumcision

Circumcision is an elective medical procedure that involves the surgical removal of the layer of skin, the foreskin, that covers the tip of the penis. The procedure is more common in the United States than in many other countries. Religious groups, including Moslems and Jews, have practiced it for centuries. Controversy exists over the medical need for circumcision. There is a very small, but definite, risk of complication from the procedure itself.

Medical reasons cited for circumcision include avoiding conditions that may require circumcision later in life, such as tightness of the foreskin, lowering the risk of infection and cancer of the penis, and cleanliness. Many physicians point to a lack of evidence for these reasons, however. It appears that circumcised infants have less risk of infections of the urinary tract than uncircumcised infants, but the risk in both groups is low.

This decision is not always easy. There are personal, emotional, and religious arguments. Medical reasons for and against circumcision are based on events that do not often occur. The procedure is uncomfortable but local anesthesia is available; it probably is more uncomfortable, or at least is remembered as such, when done at an older age. There is much written, positive and negative, about circumcision by people who often feel very strongly about their position.

Parents should talk with their physician about circumcision as early as possible and with adequate time to make an informed decision. Written material about the procedure and the care necessary for both circumcised and uncircumcised boys is available in many hospitals and from doctors' offices.

Babies at Risk

Few babies have serious problems, and help is available for those that do. All parts of the United States are included in a regional system of perinatal care that provides for special care of babies within an area. Intensive care units for babies have successfully lowered infant mortality. If a problem is suspected before birth, a mother may be told that she should deliver in a hospital with an intensive care nursery if there is not one in her community. If a problem arises without warning, the baby is stabilized and then transported by an expert team to a facility where special care is available.

Pediatricians are specialists who have been trained to recognize and treat problems in babies and children. Neonatologists are pediatricians with subspecialty training in the care of babies. Other specialists and subspecialists, such as pediatric surgeons, may be called upon for special care.

Babies with problems are usually cared for in an intensive care nursery or neonatal intensive care unit. There a baby may be placed in an incubator to keep warm, fed through a tube, or connected to a respirator to help with breathing. The baby will be monitored by specially trained nurses and complex equipment.

Neonatal intensive care units are often busy and may seem strange at first. You may feel that everyone else is taking care of your baby and there is no place for you. Be assured that the highly skilled personnel cannot take your place as a parent, and they will encourage you to be with your baby. Contact is important for both baby and parents. As soon as possible, talk to your baby and stroke him or her in the incubator. The baby needs to hear your voice and feel your touch. Soon you may be able to hold and cuddle your baby for longer periods and help with care.

Preterm Babies

The single largest problem for newborns is **preterm** birth and its complications. Premature babies are born before 37 weeks of gestation. The younger and smaller the baby is, the greater the risk of complications and the need for intensive care.

Preterm babies look different than term babies in many ways. They may appear red and skinny because they have little fat under their skin and blood vessels are close to the surface. Babies grow and develop in utero, so the more premature a baby is, the less developed it

Facts About Preterm Birth

- Across the United States 6–8% of babies are born early, but some populations have a higher risk. Preterm delivery is considered to be the single most important problem of pregnancy.
- Preterm babies can have breathing problems, brain hemorrhage, infection, and intestinal problems.
- Medical care has reduced the loss of preterm babies: the 1988 death rate for preterm newborns in the United States was 9.9 per 1,000 live births; in 1940 it was 47 per 1,000.
- The rates of preterm birth and low birth weight have not changed. The medical profession and parents must work together to improve medical and life style factors.

is. This lack of development can lead, for example, to breathing difficulties manifested as a disease called ***respiratory distress syndrome (RDS)***, feeding problems, or increased risk of infection.

Growth Retardation

Being smaller than expected for the amount of time spent in the uterus is known as intrauterine growth retardation. It is fairly common and can have a number of causes. In many situations, it is possible to detect or at least suspect this problem before birth. When prenatal care gives advance notice of intrauterine growth retardation, treatment can be started earlier.

Postmaturity

Postterm babies, those born after 42 weeks of gestation, often have problems that term babies do not. These babies are referred to as postmature. One problem is that the placenta may be less able to take care of the baby's nutritional and other needs. The baby may appear to have lost weight and be less able to meet the stress of birth.

Infection

An infection can be passed from the mother to the fetus during pregnancy or to the baby as it is born. Although both the mother and the baby have natural resistance to infection and can fight it when it occurs, some agents can cross the placenta and infect the fetus in the uterus. Good health maintenance before conception, including being immunized and avoiding being exposed to infection, can help to prevent and decrease the risk of infection before birth (see Chapter 12).

Only a small number of babies become infected during or after birth. Hospitals have policies designed to lower the risk of spreading of infection. The hospital staff will examine your baby for signs of infection. They or your doctor can give you advice on ways to decrease the risk of infection, such as good hand-washing, cord care, feeding practices, and avoiding people with obvious infections.

Going Home

If there are no complications, many babies and mothers go home 24 hours or so after birth, while they are still in a process of recovery and adjustment. The first days at home should be quiet, with extra help available if possible. Unfortunately, parental leave is not given to all parents of newborns, and not all parents have outside support to make this time easier.

Babies are very sensitive and need some time to adjust without being overly exposed to multiple sounds, intense light, or handling by many people. Allow a week for infant and maternal adjustment. Keep trips and visits from friends short. Use this time to begin to develop a routine for you and your baby.

Pediatric care for your baby is best arranged before birth. Speak with friends and health professionals about the choices in your community and select a source that meets the needs of your family. Pediatricians often like to meet mothers and fathers before the birth of the first child.

The first follow-up visit for your baby is best arranged before leaving the hospital. The timing depends on how long you were in the hospital, whether any special problems (like jaundice) need monitoring, and the practice in your local area. A visit in 1 month is common, with earlier visits recommended in many areas.

Families today come in traditional and nontraditional forms. In any family with a birth, the focus is on the mother–infant relationship. However, the social network can also include the father, siblings, relatives, and friends. All contribute to the life and growth of the infant. All are affected by the birth. All are important.

Some babies will adapt easily to their new environment, while others will struggle to maintain their composure. Much of the challenge of parenting in the first days and weeks centers on learning how to read the signals of this special and unique child. Parents must respond to signals of hunger and a need for sleep or attention and begin to build a relationship of trust that gives the baby security to grow into a healthy, competent, and confident child.

Questions to Consider...

- How can I locate a pediatrician? When should I make my first appointment?
- What was my baby's Apgar score?
- If my baby is a boy and I want him circumcised, when is the best time to do so?
- Does my baby need any special care?
- What are some good resources—books and classes—for learning basic baby care skills?

Chapter 15

After You Go Home

Beginning parenthood can be an exciting yet frustrating time. There are changes in your body, your emotions, your relationships with friends and relatives, and in the way you live your life.

The adjustment from being pregnant to being a mother begins during the first few days after delivery. It is often hard to believe that childbirth is over and that this new baby is really yours! Very often your focus is not completely on the baby, but on what happened during labor and delivery. You want to talk about it, share it, and relive it in your mind.

As you leave the hospital and begin a new routine at home, you will develop the skills that you need to care for your infant. This is often an anxious time as you wonder whether you will be able to do everything it takes to be a good mother. Tasks that you once did with ease may seem more complicated. Relax and remember that you are not born with these skills. They are learned, and it takes time.

Being aware of what is happening to your body and your emotions can help prepare you to face calmly the ups and downs of the first few months of being a new mother. You will feel the strain of labor, and it will take a while to regain your stamina. It is especially important to take care of your physical and mental well-being. A proper diet and daily exercise will increase your energy level and help you get back in shape.

As you resume your daily life, you will be faced with decisions about returning to work, child care, and family planning. Your partner and others who are important to you can help you adjust to your new role.

Your Changing Body

While you were pregnant, changes in your body and the growth of the fetus took place gradually over a 9-month period. Now that your baby has been born, your body will return to its prepregnancy state much more rapidly, but it will take some time to return to normal.

Uterus

After delivery, your uterus is hard and round and can be felt around your navel. It weighs about 2 1/2 pounds. Six weeks later, it weighs

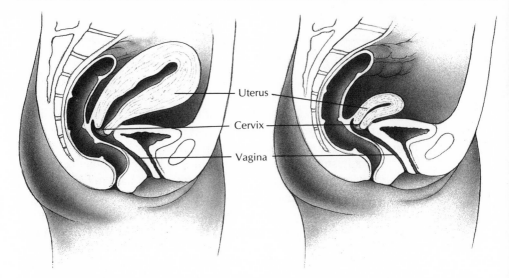

Just after birth, the uterus measures about 7 inches long and weighs about 2 pounds (left). *It can be felt just below the navel. In 6 weeks* (right) *it has returned to its normal size of about 3 inches long, weighing about 2 ounces.*

only 2 ounces and can no longer be felt by pressing on your abdomen. The opening of the uterus—the cervix—decreases to the size of a dime within 1 week of delivery.

Lochia

The vaginal discharge that occurs after delivery is called *lochia*. It consists mostly of blood and what remains of the uterine lining that was needed during pregnancy. For the first few days after delivery, the discharge is bright red, perhaps with a few small clots. The flow becomes darker and decreases, although the bright red flow may resume on occasion (ie, after breast-feeding). In about 10–14 days, the discharge becomes white or yellow and gradually stops. The length of time of the discharge differs for each woman. Tampons may be used or not, depending on whether they feel comfortable.

Return of Menstrual Periods

Your menstrual period will return in about 7–9 weeks after delivery if you are not breast-feeding. Your periods may be shorter or longer than they were before your pregnancy, but they will gradually return to what is normal for you. If you are breast-feeding, your periods may not return for several months, perhaps not until you stop breast-feeding. Your ovaries may begin to function before you have your period, however. This means that you can ovulate and become pregnant even before your menstrual period returns. Contraception should be started by 3–4 weeks after delivery if you do not want to get pregnant right away.

Perineum

The area between your vagina and rectum, called the *perineum*, stretched during delivery. You may also have had an *episiotomy* to avoid tearing during delivery, and this area must now heal. Over the weeks after the birth, these muscles will begin to regain some of their tone. You can help this process along by doing Kegel exercises. These simple exercises (described in Chapter 9) can be done anytime and anywhere. They can be started as soon as you feel comfortable enough to do them.

Abdomen

Many women are surprised and disappointed that their abdomens are flabby after delivery, making them look as if they are still pregnant. During pregnancy, the abdominal muscles stretch, and return of good muscle tone takes some time. You can do some simple exercises that will help tighten the muscles (see "Exercise" in this chapter). You may have a tendency to get a backache until the abdominal muscles tighten up and once again work with your back muscles to help you maintain an erect posture.

Discomforts

After delivery, you may find that there are times when you are physically uncomfortable. Most of these discomforts don't last and can be relieved.

Afterbirth Pains

Afterbirth pains are caused by the uterus contracting and relaxing as it returns to its normal state. The contractions are generally mild with first babies and stronger with subsequent babies and with nursing, but they last only a few days. Try changing your position, lying on your stomach with a pillow under your abdomen, and keeping your bladder empty. Your doctor may prescribe medication to help you feel more comfortable.

Painful Episiotomy

Cold packs applied immediately after delivery often lessen the discomfort of an episiotomy. Later on, cold packs or a warm sitz bath (sitting for a short time in warm water) can also make you more comfortable and help the healing process. In the hospital, you will be taught how to clean the area to prevent infection.

Hemorrhoids

Hemorrhoids can protrude or become swollen and painful during pregnancy, labor, and delivery. Sprays, ointments, or dry or moist heat (as for an episiotomy) can provide some relief. Cold witch hazel compresses are also very soothing. The hemorrhoids will gradually decrease in size and may even disappear.

Constipation

Reduced movement through the intestines and relaxed abdominal muscles often contribute to postdelivery constipation. Fear of having a bowel movement because of the pain from an episiotomy or hemorrhoids may add to the problem. A diet high in fiber and plenty of fluids and juices can help.

Breast Engorgement

You may have fullness and discomfort in your breasts 2–4 days after delivery. A well-fitting support bra will help. Ice packs may be

Warning Signs

After delivery, you should continue to watch for any abnormal changes in your health. Call your doctor if you notice any of the following symptoms:

- Fever over 100.4°F (38°C)
- Nausea and vomiting
- Painful urination, burning, and urgency (sudden, strong desire to urinate)
- Bleeding heavier than your normal period
- Pain, swelling, and tenderness in legs
- Chest pain and cough
- Hot, tender breast
- Persistent perineal pain with increasing tenderness

applied to relieve the discomfort. If you are not nursing, you should not empty, stimulate, or pump your breasts; this will only cause more milk to be produced. The discomfort should disappear in about 36 hours and can be relieved by pain medications.

Breast-Feeding

Almost every woman can produce milk after her baby is born, and almost every woman can breast-feed successfully. Still, breast-feeding may not be for all women. Many factors are involved in each woman's decision: life style, desire, attitude, and time. If bottle-feeding is chosen, the baby can be well nourished with formula. If you use only bottle-feeding, however, your milk supply will dry up, and breast-feeding will no longer be an option.

In addition to exclusive use of either method, there are combinations of feeding schedules from which you can choose:

- Breast-feeding with no bottles for the first 6 months
- Breast-feeding for a short time, such as 6 weeks or 3 months, and then bottle-feeding
- Breast-feeding supplemented by occasional bottle-feeding
- Breast-feeding a few times a day and bottle-feeding a few times a day

Some women are reluctant to try to breast-feed. Usually, misinformation or lack of information is the cause. For instance, the amount of milk made for the baby does not depend on the size or shape of a woman's breasts. Nor does nipple size or shape affect the ability to nurse.

If you did not breast-feed other children, it does not mean you cannot breast-feed the new baby. If you were not successful breast-

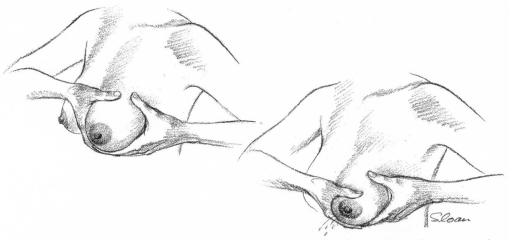

To manually express milk, massage the breast, working evenly around each one toward the nipple. With thumb and forefinger about an inch from the nipple, press in and up to release the milk. Do not squeeze the nipple itself—this will close the ducts.

feeding before, a few simple changes in technique will often make a difference. Although breast-feeding is the natural way to feed a baby, it still involves learning and practice.

If you plan to return to school or work after the birth, you can breast-feed, too. Some mothers combine formula feeding with a decrease in the frequency of breast-feeding to a few times a day. Other women may collect milk from their breasts either manually or with a pump before going to school or work. They leave the milk with the baby's caretaker during the day.

Breast-feeding is not for every woman. Women who have infections that could be passed to the baby or who are taking certain drugs should not breast-feed. If you are taking medication, you should check with your doctor about whether it might affect the baby if you breast-feed. The levels of most drugs in breast milk are so low that they have no effect on the baby.

A mother who chooses not to or who is unable to breast-feed should not feel guilty. Your baby can be well nourished and thrive with baby formula. Bottle-feeding does require more care and preparation than breast-feeding, however. Everything used in the feeding of formula—from the bottles and nipples to the brushes used to clean them—must be well cleaned and sterilized before each feeding. The formula must be prepared exactly according to the directions. Formula that is too weak or too strong is not good for the baby.

Bottle-feeding costs more than breast-feeding. In addition to the formula, all the bottles, nipples, and bottle brushes must be bought.

However, any woman who would like to bottle-feed can often find financial help to do so. A government program called Women, Infants, and Children (WIC) provides formula for mothers who cannot afford it.

Using prepared formulas can allow others to help with the feeding. This is handy for the mother who wants to return to work outside the home soon after birth. It also lets others in the family, such as the father and other children, share in feeding the infant.

If you decide against breast-feeding, your breasts may be sore, feel very full, and leak for a few days. A good support bra, good personal hygiene, and application of ice packs will relieve the discomfort until your breasts return to their prepregnancy state.

Baby Blues and Postpartum Depression

It is very common for new mothers to feel sad, afraid, angry, or anxious after childbirth. Most new mothers have these feelings in a mild form called postpartum blues, baby blues, or maternity blues. Instead of this relatively mild sadness and anxiety, a few new mothers develop a more serious condition called postpartum depression. This condition lasts longer, is more intense, and may require counseling and treatment.

Blues or Depression?

Many new mothers are surprised at how fragile, alone, and overwhelmed they feel after the birth of a child. Their feelings don't seem to match their expectations. They wonder, "What have I got to be depressed about?" They fear that these feelings somehow mean that they are bad mothers.

In fact, about 70% of women have the baby blues after childbirth. Feelings of depression, anxiety, and anger usually begin about 3 days after birth. At this time, new mothers may feel sad and weepy, anxious, and moody. For no clear reason, they may feel angry at the new baby, their partner, or at their other children. They may cry unexpectedly. Sometimes they have trouble sleeping, eating, and making decisions. They almost always question whether they are able to handle the important new responsibility of caring for a baby.

As bewildering and frightening as these thoughts and feelings seem at the time, the baby blues usually last only for a short time—a few hours to a week or so—and go away without the need for treatment.

Some women develop postpartum depression, which is marked by more intense feelings of sadness, anxiety, or despair that disrupt the new mother's ability to function. If not recognized and treated, postpartum depression may become worse or may last longer than it needs to. There are a number of signs and symptoms of postpartum depression:

- Baby blues that don't go away after 2 weeks, or strong feelings of depression and anger that begin to surface a month or two after childbirth
- Feelings of sadness, doubt, guilt, helplessness, or hopelessness that seem to increase with each week and begin to disrupt a woman's normal functioning
- Not being able to sleep even when tired, or sleeping most of the time, even when the baby is awake
- Marked changes in appetite
- Extreme concern and worry about the baby, or lack of interest in or feelings for the baby or other members of her family
- Anxiety or panic attacks
- Fear of harming the baby or thoughts of self-harm

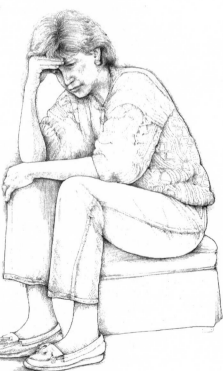

If you have any of these signs of postpartum depression, you should discuss this with your doctor and take steps right away to get the support and help you need.

Periods of sadness, fear, anger, and anxiety after childbirth are quite common and do not mean that you are a failure as a woman or as a mother, or that you are mentally ill. They do mean that you and your body are adjusting to the hormonal and other changes that follow the birth of a child. Blues that don't go away after a few weeks may be a sign of a more serious depression. If your feelings do not lessen after a few weeks and begin to interfere with your functioning, contact your doctor.

Return to Daily Living

Bringing home a new baby is a special time for both you and your partner. But sometimes you may feel moments of panic. If you try to keep in mind that your relationship with each other will be changed, that your patterns of daily living will be new, and that old routines may no longer work, you will be able to begin your new family life at home feeling much more relaxed. This does not mean that things will not be as good as or even better than before, just that they will be very different.

A new baby touches the lives of the entire family. Each member has a role and should be encouraged to become involved in the baby's care. One of the best things to do is talk—to your partner, your parents, your friends, and to other mothers. Share your concerns and listen to those of the important people in your life.

Mother and Baby

First-time mothers often believe that they should automatically know how to care for a newborn. In fact, new mothers need to learn mothering skills just as they learn any other important life skill. It takes time and patience.

Some mothers are burdened by notions of having a perfect baby and being a perfect mother. Babies have distinct personalities from birth—some are simply easier to care for than others. If a mother thinks she is not living up to the "perfect mother" ideal, whether it is her own or that of her friends or parents, she may suffer from feelings of inadequacy and depression.

In reality, no mother is perfect. Most women find juggling the responsibilities of a new baby with household duties, other children, and a job to be extremely demanding, even if they have a lot of emotional and financial support.

Fatigue is common during the first weeks postpartum. Rest—or lack of it—will be one of the most important factors in your new life. It is often difficult to get enough rest because of the baby's erratic schedule. Try to sleep when the baby sleeps. Do not use this time to catch up on chores. If you have an older child, try to arrange for quiet entertainment while you and the baby rest. Although everyone will want to visit and see the new baby, try to limit visitors. There will be plenty of time to show off the baby when you feel comfortable and well rested.

Don't hesitate to accept offers of help from your family, partner, and friends. Often people who offer to help don't know what they can or should do for you, or what will help you the most. Be specific—ask a friend to bring a casserole for dinner, to stop at the grocery store, to drop off laundry, or to watch the baby or older child for 2 hours so that you can rest.

Include labor savers in your budget. Use a diaper service or disposable diapers. Use prepared formula if you are not breast-feeding. Hire someone to clean the house. It is more important for you to get the rest you need than that the housework be done to your usual standards.

Father

A new father's needs and concerns often are not given the attention they deserve and require. Much of the advice fathers receive is related to how to help the mother, but adjusting to the presence of a new baby in the home can be just as difficult for him. The father may also have ambivalent feelings about parenthood. He may throw himself into work or start spending time away from home. Or he may find himself fully engrossed in fatherhood.

A father's bonding with his new child can be greatly enhanced by his participation in the care of the baby. A new mother may find it hard to let someone else care for the baby at first, more because of her own concerns about doing everything right than because she doubts the father's ability to take care of the baby. It is very important that the father hold and care for the baby and get to know his son or daughter.

Siblings

Older children often have feelings of jealousy and uncertainty about the new baby. They may express these feelings in a variety of attention-getting ways. If a baby gets so much attention, then the older child may act like a baby. He or she may show anger toward the mother for paying so much attention to the baby, or toward the baby itself.

The arrival at home of a younger brother or sister is a difficult time for an older child. It is a good time for the father to start developing (or strengthening) a close relationship with the older child. It is

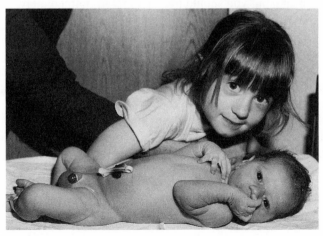

Photo by Marjorie M. Pyle, RNC, ACCE

not a good idea to send an older child to stay with someone else for a while. Instead, ask a relative or friend to stay with you and to pay extra attention to the needs of the older child.

Grandparents

Grandparents respond in many different ways to the birth of a grand-child. They may hold back, not wanting to interfere. They may give lots of advice, although they may not intend it as interference.

If grandparents are coming to stay and help, set a date for their return home. If there are problems or disagreements, it is important that the new parents make the decisions and that they back up each other in these decisions.

Exercise

Daily exercise can help restore muscle strength and return your body to its prepregnancy shape. It can actually help decrease fatigue and increase your energy level and your general sense of well-being.

If you had a cesarean delivery, a complicated birth, or postpartum complications, check with your doctor before beginning an exercise program. Otherwise, start when you feel up to it. Follow the same general guidelines as you did when you were pregnant (see Chapter 7).

If you didn't exercise during pregnancy, start slowly with easy exercises and gradually build up to more difficult ones. If you exercised regularly throughout the pregnancy, you have a head start on getting back into shape, but you should not try to return immediately to the level and intensity of exercise you did before the birth.

Walking is a good way to return to an exercise program. Brisk walks several times a week will prepare you to do more strenuous exercise when you feel up to it. Swimming is also an excellent postpartum exercise.

You will want to design your own exercise program to meet your own needs. This program can include improving your heart and lungs, toning your muscles, or both. Your doctor can recommend types of exercises for you. There are also specially designed postpartum exercise classes that you can join.

Nutrition and Diet

You will lose about 18–20 pounds within 10 days after delivery. It is tempting to try to lose more so that you can wear your prepregnancy clothes again. Be patient. It is best to lose about 1/2 pound per week. If you continue to eat the well-balanced diet that you began in pregnancy, in an amount appropriate for your body weight, you will return to your normal weight within 2 months of delivery. Coupling this diet with exercises found elsewhere in this chapter will keep your muscles in tone.

If you are breast-feeding, you need extra fluid, calories, calcium, and protein. A nursing mother needs the foods normally required for her own body plus extra food to produce milk for her baby—about 600 more calories a day than she needed before pregnancy. It is easy to add the extra food needed for nursing if you are already eating a well-balanced diet made up of a variety of foods from each of the four food groups (see Chapter 8).

Calcium, which is particularly important for nursing mothers, is supplied by milk used as a drink or in cooking, and by yogurt, cheese, cottage cheese, ice cream, and ice milk. If you cannot tolerate milk products, other sources of calcium can be suggested by your doctor. You should avoid nicotine, alcohol, and other drugs that can have a damaging effect on your baby.

Work

There are a number of factors to consider in deciding whether and when to resume working after the birth of your baby, and there are a variety of options from which you can choose. Your doctor may recommend that you remain at home for a certain period of time to recover your strength before returning to work.

Financial factors should be considered, of course, as well as the cost and availability of child care. If you are breast-feeding, you may have to wean your baby or cut down the number of feedings before you return to work full time. Breast milk can be saved to be given to the baby later if you can't be there.

Employers are becoming more flexible and offering more options to working mothers. Many women work part time or even share one full-time job. With home computers (and copiers and fax machines), some women find that they can comfortably work at home.

Sex

Before you have sexual intercourse, you should wait until the healing process is complete to avoid hurting delicate tissues. Sexual intercourse can usually be resumed when your pelvic structures and the episiotomy are healed and you feel comfortable. This usually takes

Postpartum Exercises

Leg Slides

This simple exercise tones abdominal and leg muscles. It does not put much strain on your incision if you have had a cesarean birth. You should try to repeat this exercise several times a day.

- Lie flat on your back and bend your knees slightly.
- Inhale, slide your right leg from a bent to a straight position, exhale, and bend it back again.
- Be sure that you keep both feet on the floor and keep them relaxed.
- Repeat with your left leg.

Head Lifts

Head lifts can progress to shoulder lifts and curl-ups, all of which strengthen the abdominal muscles. When you feel comfortable doing 10 head lifts at a time, proceed to shoulder lifts.

- Lie on your back with your arms along your sides. Bend your knees so that your feet are flat on the floor.
- Inhale and relax your abdomen.
- Exhale slowly as you lift your head off the floor.
- Inhale as you lower your head again.

Shoulder Lifts

Begin the same way as you would for head lifts. When you feel comfortable doing 10 shoulder lifts at a time, proceed to curl-ups.

- Inhale and relax your abdomen.
- Exhale slowly and lift your head and shoulders off the floor. Reach with your arms so that you don't use them for support.
- Inhale as you lower your shoulders to the floor.

Curl-ups

Begin the same way as you would for head lifts, lying on your back with your knees bent and your arms at your sides. Keep your lower back flat on the floor.

- Inhale, relaxing your abdomen.
- Exhale. Reach with your arms, and slowly raise your torso to the point halfway between your knees and the floor (about a 45° angle).
- Inhale as you lower yourself to the floor.

Kneeling Pelvic Tilt

Tilting your pelvis back toward your spine helps strengthen your abdominal muscles.

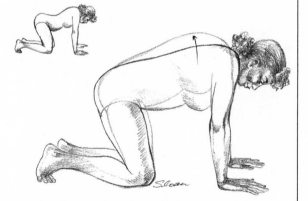

- Begin on your hands and knees. Your back should be relaxed, not curved or arched.
- Inhale.
- Exhale and pull your buttocks forward, rotating the pubic bone upward.
- Hold for a count of three, then inhale and relax.
- Repeat five times and add one or two repetitions a day if you can.

Child Care Options

A baby may be cared for in the parents' home or at another location. For care in the home, contact employment agencies specializing in child care professionals. This private care is very expensive, however. You may wish to place your child in a day care center or in the home of a licensed provider or a relative. Your pediatrician can be a good source of information on child care. Here are some points to consider in selecting child care:

- Gather information about the available centers. Find out where they are located, what the hours of operation are, and the cost of care.
- Visit the center. Be sure to go more than once. Make an appointment the first time, and then drop in unannounced. See what the physical setting is like. Observe the children who are there. Find out what a typical daily schedule is and what is typically served to the children at meal and snack times. Be sure the facilities are well equipped and large enough to handle the number of children, and that there are enough care providers present (one adult per three to four infants, four to five toddlers, or six to nine preschoolers).
- Check credentials. When you leave your child in the hands of a professional, you should know something about that person's background and priorities. If the person is licensed or registered with the local government, ask to see the document. If there are any written policies concerning philosophy, procedures, or discipline, be sure to get copies. Find out if the care provider has had training in first aid, if he or she is willing to give your child prescribed medications, and what plans are in place in case of a medical emergency. If possible, get recommendations from others who have used the center or care provider.

about 3–4 weeks. It is important for you and your partner to discuss this beforehand with your doctor and with each other so that there will be few misunderstandings and frustrations later.

When you think you are ready to resume sexual relations, proceed slowly and gently. Try to choose a time when you are not rushed. You may notice a dryness of the vagina. This decreased lubrication is a normal response of your body. It may last as long as you breast-feed or until your first menstrual period. Use a water-soluble cream or jelly, baby oil, or saliva to provide lubrication during this time.

Sometimes you may not be as interested in sex as you were before you gave birth. Fatigue is often the major cause of a lack of

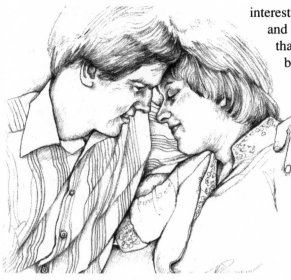

interest in sex at this time for both men and women. You may also be afraid that intercourse will be painful because you have had an episiotomy or that you will become pregnant. For your comfort, you and your partner may want to try different sexual positions.

The emotional turmoil caused by the changing roles of both new parents may cause a loss of interest in sex as new roles are learned. The constant presence and demands of the baby may decrease your desire.

If there are difficulties, it is important to talk about them. Spend time together without the baby at least once or twice a week. Try to avoid talking about the baby and the household at these special times. Talk about yourselves and each other. Rediscover what brought you together in the first place. There are other forms of sharing your sexual feelings—stroking, touching, or cuddling—that can be very satisfying.

Family Planning

Once you and your partner decide to resume intercourse, you must also decide how you wish to space your children. For most women, at least 11/2 to 2 years between births is best. You should choose some form of birth control before you have intercourse for the first time.

There are many methods of birth control available. Because there are advantages to each method, it is best to discuss them thoroughly with your doctor and your partner so that you can select a method that meets your needs. Here are some things you might want to consider:

• Effectiveness of the method
• How comfortable you feel using the method
• General health of you and your partner
• Risks involved in the method
• Cost
• Convenience of use

Any method of contraception can be effective in protecting against unwanted pregnancy if it is used carefully, correctly, and consistently. To work properly, contraception should be used at all times, exactly according to instructions. For this reason, you should give serious thought to selecting a method you will feel comfortable using on a regular basis.

The birth control pill and the intrauterine device (IUD) are the most effective methods of temporary or reversible contraception. This is largely because these methods are always in your body and act continuously to prevent pregnancy. Other techniques must be used each time you have intercourse. Still others are surgical procedures that should be considered permanent once they are performed.

Birth Control Pills

The most popular method of contraception is the birth control pill, or oral contraceptive, which contains synthetic female hormones that closely resemble those your body produces naturally. When you take the pill as prescribed, your body stops ovulating or releasing eggs, but you still have a monthly period. Because there is no egg available to be fertilized, pregnancy cannot occur.

Intrauterine Device

The intrauterine device (IUD) is a small plastic device (sometimes containing copper or hormones) that is inserted in and left inside the uterus. The presence of the IUD in the uterus creates a reaction that prevents the sperm from fertilizing the egg in the tubes.

Intrauterine device (IUD)

Barrier Methods

Barrier methods of contraception prevent the sperm from gaining access to the female reproductive system and fertilizing the egg:

• The diaphragm is a round rubber dome that fits inside the woman's vagina and covers her cervix. (If you used a diaphragm previously, you must be remeasured after the birth of your baby.)

- The cervical cap works similarly to a diaphragm and can remain in place longer.
- The condom is a thin rubber sheath worn by the man over his erect penis.
- The vaginal sponge is a small plastic sponge containing spermicide that is inserted in the upper part of the vagina.
- Spermicides contain a chemical that kills sperm and are placed in the vagina close to the cervix.

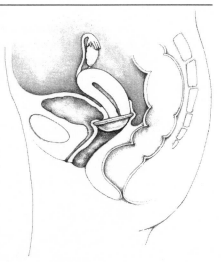

Diaphragm

These barrier methods must be used each time you have intercourse to be effective. The exception is the vaginal sponge, which can be retained in the vagina for up to 24 hours, regardless of how often you have intercourse. Barrier methods are often used in combination with each other to provide a twofold contraceptive effect.

Periodic Abstinence

Also referred to as natural family planning, periodic abstinence involves avoiding sexual intercourse during those times in your menstrual cycle when your chances of becoming pregnant are greatest. By using one of the methods designed to calculate when ovulation is expected, you and your partner know when to abstain from sexual relations to avoid the possibility of a live sperm reaching and fertilizing a mature egg. Your doctor can provide you with information about the four ways of determining when ovulation is likely to occur:

- Basal body temperature method
- Mucus method
- Symptothermal method
- Calendar method

Sterilization

If you and your partner decide that you definitely don't want to have any more children, sterilization is a means of permanent birth control. It does not guarantee sterility, although more than 99% of women who are sterilized do not become pregnant. Sterilization is popular because it frees a couple from the need to use birth control methods.

Sterilization of a woman is called ***tubal ligation***. It involves either cutting or placing a band or clip around the fallopian tubes, blocking the sperm from reaching and fertilizing the egg. A man is sterilized by ***vasectomy***, in which the vas deferens, the tubes through which sperm travels, are sealed so that sperm cannot be released during climax. Both procedures can be done at any time, usually on an outpatient basis. Women often choose to have sterilization postpartum while they are still in the hospital. It can be done more easily at this time because the still-enlarged uterus pushes the fallopian tubes up so they can be sealed through a small incision in your navel.

Fallopian tube

During postpartum sterilization, a small vertical or horizontal cut is made below the navel, and each fallopian tube is pulled through the incision (above). *A section of the tube is closed off with surgical thread, and the section between the ties is removed* (right).

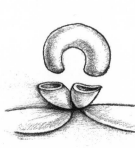

As is true of any operation, sterilization has some risks. Serious problems can and do happen in about 1 in every 1,000 women who have the operation. Most of the time they can be treated and corrected.

Although there is a slight chance of becoming pregnant after sterilization, as well as a slight chance that the operation could be reversed, a sterilization operation should be considered permanent. You and your partner must be certain you do not want any more chil-

During a vasectomy, one or two small cuts are made in the skin of the scrotum. Each vas is pulled through the opening until it forms a loop. A small section is cut out of the loop and removed.

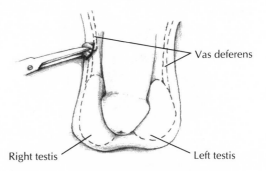

Vas deferens

Right testis   Left testis

dren—now or in the future. If for any reason you may want to have children in the future, you may wish to consider a different form of birth control.

Breast-Feeding and Family Planning

Ovulation and menstruation often do not occur while nursing. Thus, the risk of pregnancy is decreased for a woman who breast-feeds compared with one who does not breast-feed. Breast-feeding should not be considered a form of birth control, however. Ovulation can occur before you begin to menstruate again after pregnancy. If you don't use birth control, you could become pregnant, even if you are breast-feeding.

Birth control pills may be used while you are breast-feeding. They may cause a slight decrease in the amount of milk you produce, but this shouldn't pose a problem.

Follow-up Visit

You should make an appointment to visit your doctor 4–6 weeks after the birth of your baby. Your weight, blood pressure, breasts, and abdomen will be checked, and you will be given a pelvic exam. Your doctor will determine how well your body has recovered from the changes you have gone through and will be able to tell if there are any problems.

You should also discuss any questions or concerns you have about birth control, sexual difficulties, or emotional problems. This is the best time to resolve any problems you may be having and to prepare for an ongoing program of health care for the future.

*Your doctor can answer any questions you might
have, and can help you plan your routine care
postpartum.*

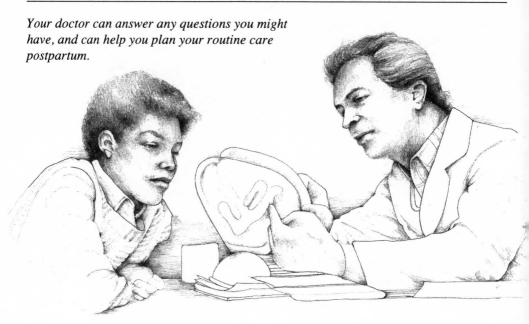

Questions to Consider...

- Is my body to returning to normal on time?
- If I'm breast-feeding, can I take any medications to relieve discomforts?
- Should I receive counseling for postpartum depression?
- Am I trying to do too much and not getting enough rest?
- Should I be exercising or changing my diet?
- How can I locate child care?
- When can my partner and I resume sex?
- What form of family planning is best for me?

Appendix A

Personal Pregnancy Diary

MY HEALTH CARE TEAM

Obstetricians' names:

_____

_____

_____

Obstetricians' address:

_____

_____

_____

Nursing staff:

_____

_____

_____

Telephone/answering service:

Day_____

Night_____

Hospital_____

Receptionist:_____

Pediatrician's name:

_____

Address:_____

_____

_____

Telephone/answering service:

_____

_____

_____

MY CHILDBIRTH EDUCATION

Educator:_____

Place: _____

_____

_____

Beginning date:_____

Ending date:_____

Telephone:_____

FIRST SIGNS

I first heard my baby's heartbeat:_____Date I first felt my baby move:_____

MEDICATIONS

Medications Taken	Dose	Date Started	Date Ended

Allergies:_____

_____

VITAL STATISTICS

My prepregnant weight:_____lbs.   Last menstrual period:_____

My blood type:_____ Rh factor: _____Rubella status:_____

SPECIAL TESTS

Date	Procedure	Findings

PRENATAL VISITS

Visit	Date	Weeks	Weight	Blood Pressure	Uterus Height (cm)	Questions/Comments
1st						
2nd						
3rd						
4th						
5th						
6th						
7th						
8th						
9th						
10th						
11th						
12th						
13th						

LABOR AND DELIVERY

Support person:_____

My due date:_____ My labor began:_____

My baby was born:_____ Time of delivery:_____

Delivery by:_____

My baby's weight:_____ Length:_____

Hospital where my baby was born:_____

_____

_____

MEDICAL RECORD

Mother: _____   Baby:_____
          (no.)   (no.)

POSTPARTUM VISITS

Mother

Date:_____Weight:_____Blood pressure:_____

Family planning:_____

Comments:_____

Baby

Date:_____Weight:_____Length:_____

Special care for my baby:_____

_____

Baby's feeding:_____

Comments:_____

_____

*This space has been reserved for the baby—
an ultrasound scan, birth announcement, or photograph*

Baby's name:_____

Date:_____

Appendix B

Medical Record

DATE _____

NAME _____
     LAST   FIRST   MIDDLE

ID # _____ HOSPITAL OF DELIVERY _____

NEWBORN'S PHYSICIAN _____ REFERRED BY _____

BIRTHDATE	AGE	RACE	MARITAL STATUS	ADDRESS:		
MO DAY YR		W B O	S M W D SEP			
OCCUPATION ☐ HOMEMAKER ☐ OUTSIDE WORK _____ ☐ STUDENT Type of Work			EDUCATION (LAST GRADE COMPLETED)	ZIP: PHONE: MEDICAID # / INSURANCE		
EMERGENCY CONTACT:					RELATIONSHIP:	PHONE:

TOTAL PREG	FULL TERM	PREMATURE	ABORTIONS INDUCED	ABORTIONS SPONTANEOUS	ECTOPICS	MULTIPLE BIRTHS	LIVING

PAST PREGNANCIES (LAST SIX)

DATE MO / YR	GA WEEKS	LENGTH OF LABOR	BIRTH WEIGHT	TYPE DELIVERY	ANES.	PLACE OF DELIVERY	PERINATAL MORTALITY YES / NO	TREATMENT PRETERM LABOR YES/NO	COMMENTS / COMPLICATIONS

PAST MEDICAL HISTORY

	O Neg + Pos.	DETAIL POSITIVE REMARKS INCLUDE DATE & TREATMENT			
DIABETES			RH SENSITIZED		
HYPERTENSION			TUBERCULOSIS		
HEART DISEASE			ASTHMA		
RHEUMATIC FEVER			ALLERGIES (DRUGS)		
MITRAL VALVE PROLAPSE			GYN SURGERY		
KIDNEY DISEASE / UTI			OPERATIONS / HOSPITALIZATIONS (YEAR & REASON)		
NERVOUS AND MENTAL			ANESTHETIC COMPLICATIONS		
EPILEPSY			HISTORY OF ABNORMAL PAP		
HEPATITIS / LIVER DISEASE			UTERINE ANOMALY		
VARICOSITIES / PHLEBITIS			INFERTILITY		
THYROID DYSFUNCTION			IN UTERO DES EXPOSURE		
MAJOR ACCIDENTS			STREET DRUGS		
HISTORY OF BLOOD TRANSFUSION			OTHER		
USE OF TOBACCO		# CIGS / DAY PRIOR TO PREG _____ # CIGS / DAY NOW _____ AGE ONSET SMOKING _____ YEARS	USE OF ALCOHOL	# DRINKS / WK PRIOR TO PREG _____ # DRINKS / WK NOW _____ AGE ONSET DRINKING _____ YEARS	

INFECTION SCREENING	YES	NO	PATIENT OR PARTNER HAVE HISTORY OF GENITAL HERPES?		
HIGH RISK AIDS?			RASH OR VIRAL ILLNESS SINCE LAST MENSTRUAL PERIOD?		
HIGH RISK HEPATITIS B?			HISTORY OF STD, GC, CHLAMYDIA, HPV, SYPHILIS?		
LIVE WITH SOMEONE WITH TB OR EXPOSED TO TB?			OTHER?		

243

GENETICS SCREENING
INCLUDES PATIENT, BABY'S FATHER, OR ANYONE IN EITHER FAMILY WITH:

	YES	NO		YES	NO
1. PATIENT'S AGE ≥ 35 YEARS?			10. HUNTINGTON CHOREA?		
2. ITALIAN, GREEK, MEDITERRANEAN, OR ORIENTAL BACKGROUND (MCV < 80)?			11. MENTAL RETARDATION?		
3. NEURAL TUBE DEFECT (MENINGOMYELOCELE, OPEN SPINE, OR ANENCEPHALY)?			IF YES, WAS PERSON TESTED FOR FRAGILE X?		
4. DOWN SYNDROME			12. OTHER INHERITED GENETIC OR CHROMOSOMAL DISORDER?		
5. JEWISH (TAY–SACHS)			13. PATIENT OR BABY'S FATHER HAD A CHILD WITH BIRTH DEFECTS NOT LISTED ABOVE, ≥ 3 FIRST-TRIMESTER SPONTANEOUS ABORTIONS, OR A STILLBIRTH?		
6. SICKLE CELL DISEASE OR TRAIT?					
7. HEMOPHILIA?			14. MEDICATIONS OR STREET DRUGS SINCE LAST MENSTRUAL PERIOD?		
8. MUSCULAR DYSTROPHY?			IF YES, AGENT(S)		
9. CYSTIC FIBROSIS?					

COMMENTS _____
_____
_____
_____

PRESENT PREGNANCY

	O Neg + Pos.	DETAIL POSITIVE REMARKS INCLUDE DATE & TYPE RX.			
1. VAGINAL BLEEDING			5. HEADACHE		
2. VAGINAL DISCHARGE / ODOR			6. ABDOMINAL PAIN		
3. VOMITING			7. URINARY COMPLAINTS		
4. CONSTIPATION			8. FEBRILE EPISODE		
			9. OTHER		

COMMENTS _____
_____

_____ INTERVIEWER'S SIGNATURE_____

INITIAL PHYSICAL EXAMINATION

DATE _____ / _____ / _____   PRE-PREGNANCY WEIGHT _____   HEIGHT _____   BP _____

1. HEENT	☐ NORMAL	☐ ABNORMAL	12. RECTUM	☐ NORMAL	☐ ABNORMAL	
2. FUNDI	☐ NORMAL	☐ ABNORMAL	13. VULVA	☐ NORMAL	☐ CONDYLOMA	☐ LESIONS
3. TEETH	☐ NORMAL	☐ ABNORMAL	14. VAGINA	☐ NORMAL	☐ INFLAMMATION	☐ DISCHARGE
4. THYROID	☐ NORMAL	☐ ABNORMAL	15. CERVIX	☐ NORMAL	☐ INFLAMMATION	☐ LESIONS
5. BREASTS	☐ NORMAL	☐ ABNORMAL	16. UTERUS	☐ NORMAL	☐ ABNORMAL	☐ FIBROIDS _____WEEKS
6. LUNGS	☐ NORMAL	☐ ABNORMAL	17. ADNEXA	☐ NORMAL	☐ MASS	
7. HEART	☐ NORMAL	☐ ABNORMAL	18. DIAGONAL CONJUGATE	☐ REACHED	☐ NO	_____ CM
8. ABDOMEN	☐ NORMAL	☐ ABNORMAL	19. SPINES	☐ AVERAGE	☐ PROMINENT	☐ BLUNT
9. EXTREMITIES	☐ NORMAL	☐ ABNORMAL	20. SACRUM	☐ CONCAVE	☐ STRAIGHT	☐ ANTERIOR
10. SKIN	☐ NORMAL	☐ ABNORMAL	21. ARCH	☐ NORMAL	☐ WIDE	☐ NARROW
11. LYMPH NODES	☐ NORMAL	☐ ABNORMAL	22. PELVIC TYPE	GYNECOID	☐ YES ☐ NO	

COMMENTS (Number and explain abnormals) _____
_____
_____
_____
_____

_____ EXAM BY: _____

Patient Addressograph

ACOG ANTEPARTUM RECORD

DATE _____

NAME _____
     LAST   FIRST   MIDDLE

ID # _____

PROBLEMS/PLANS (DRUG ALLERGY:)	MEDICATION LIST: Start date Stop date
1.	1.
2.	2.
3.	3.
4.	4.

EDD CONFIRMATION

INITIAL EDD:

LMP   ___/___/___   = EDD ___/___/___

INITIAL EXAM   ___/___/___ = ___ WKS. = EDD ___/___/___

ULTRASOUND   ___/___/___ = ___ WKS. = EDD ___/___/___

INITIAL EDD   ___/___/___   INITIALED BY _____

LMP □ DEFINITE   MENARCHE _____ (AGE ONSET)

□ NORMAL AMOUNT/DURATION   MENSES MONTHLY □ YES □ NO

□ APPROXIMATE (MONTH KNOWN)   FREQUENCY Q _____ DAYS

□ UNKNOWN   PRIOR MENSES _____ DATE

ON BCP'S AT CONCEPTION □ NO □ YES

HCG – ___/___/___   HCG + ___/___/___

18-20 WEEK EDD UPDATE:

QUICKENING   ___/___/___ + 22 WKS. = ___/___/___

FUNDAL HT. AT UMBIL.   ___/___/___ + 20 WKS. = ___/___/___

FHT W / FETOSCOPE   ___/___/___ + 20 WKS. = ___/___/___

ULTRASOUND   ___/___/___ = ___ WKS. = ___/___/___

FINAL EDD   ___/___/___   INITIALED BY _____

32-34 WEEK EDD - UTERINE SIZE CONCORDANCE

± 4 OR MORE CM SUGGESTS THE NEED FOR ULTRASOUND EVALUATION

VISIT DATE (YEAR_____)												
WEEKS GEST. BEST EST.												
HT FUNDUS (CM)												
PRESENTATION - VTX, BR, TRANSVERSE												
FHR PRESENT: F=FETOSCOPE O=ABSENT D=DOPTONE												
FETAL MOVEMENT: +=PRESENT D=DECREASED O=ABSENT												
PREMATURITY: SIGNS/SYMPTOMS: VAGINAL BLEEDING												
MUCUS SHOW / DISCHARGE												
+ PRESENT CRAMPS / CONTRACTIONS												
O ABSENT DYSURIA												
PELVIC PRESSURE												
CERVIX EXAM (DIL./EFF./STA.)												
BLOOD PRESSURE INITIAL												
REPEAT												
EDEMA + PRESENT O ABSENT												
WEIGHT												
CUMULATIVE WEIGHT GAIN												
URINE: (GLUCOSE/ALBUMIN/KETONES)												
NEXT APPOINTMENT												
PROVIDER												
TEST REMINDERS	8-18 WEEKS CVS/AMNIO/MSAFP			24-28 WEEKS GLUCOSE SCREEN/RhIG								

GUIDELINES: EDUCATION AND LABORATORY

INITIAL LABS	DATE	RESULT	REVIEWED	COMMENTS / ADDITIONAL LAB
BLOOD TYPE	/ /	A B AB O		
RH TYPE	/ /	+ / −		
ANTIBODY SCREEN	/ /	− / +		
HCT / HGB	/ /	_____ % _____ g/dl		
PAP SMEAR	/ /	NORMAL / ABNORMAL / _____		
RUBELLA	/ /	− / +		
VDRL	/ /	− / +		
GC	/ /	− / +		
URINE CULTURE / SCREEN	/ /	− / +		
HB S AG	/ /	− / +		

8 - 18 WEEK LABS (WHEN INDICATED)	DATE	RESULT		
ULTRASOUND	/ /			
MSAFP	/ /	_____ MOM		
AMNIO / CVS	/ /	− / +		
KARYOTYPE	/ /	46, XX OR 46, XY / OTHER _____		
ALPHA-FETOPROTEIN	/ /	NORMAL _____ ABNORMAL _____		

24 - 28 WEEK LABS (WHEN INDICATED)	DATE	RESULT		
HCT / HGB	/ /	_____ % _____ g/dl		
DIABETES SCREEN	/ /	1 HR. _____		
GTT (IF SCREEN ABNORMAL)	/ /	___ FBS ___ 1 HR. ___ 2 HR. ___ 3 HR.		
RH ANTIBODY SCREEN	/ /	− / +		
Rhig GIVEN (28 WKS)	/ /	SIGNATURE _____		

32 - 36 WEEK LABS (WHEN INDICATED)	DATE	RESULT		
ULTRASOUND	/ /	− / +		
VDRL	/ /	− / +		
GC	/ /	− / +		
HCT / HGB	/ /	_____ % _____ g/dl		

OPTIONAL LAB (HIGH RISK GROUPS)	DATE	RESULT		
HIV	/ /			
HGB ELECTROPHORESIS	/ /	AA AS SS AC SC AF		
CHLAMYDIA	/ /	− / +		

PLANS / EDUCATION

COUNSELED
YES   NO

TOXOPLASMOSIS PRECAUTIONS (CATS / RAW MEAT)_____
CHILDBIRTH CLASSES_____
PHYSICAL ACTIVITY_____
PREMATURE LABOR SIGNS_____
NUTRITION COUNSELING_____
METHOD OF ANESTHESIA_____
BREAST OR BOTTLE FEEDING_____
NEWBORN CAR SEAT_____
POSTPARTUM BIRTH CONTROL_____
ENVIRONMENTAL / WORK HAZARDS_____

COUNSELED
YES   NO

TUBAL STERILIZATION_____
VBAC COUNSELING_____
CIRCUMCISION_____
TRAVEL _____

REQUESTS _____

OTHER _____

TUBAL STERILIZATION   DATE   INITIALS
CONSENT SIGNED   ___ / ___ / ___   _____

Glossary

Abruptio Placentae: A condition in which the placenta separates from the inner wall of the uterus before the baby is born.

Alpha-fetoprotein (AFP): A protein produced by the fetus that is present in amniotic fluid and in the mother's blood.

Amenorrhea: The absence of menstrual periods.

Amniocentesis: A procedure in which a small amount of amniotic fluid is taken from the sac surrounding the fetus and tested.

Amniotic Fluid: Water in the sac surrounding the fetus in the mother's uterus.

Analgesia: Relief of pain without total loss of sensation.

Anencephaly: A type of neural tube defect that occurs when the fetus's head and brain do not develop normally.

Anesthesia: Relief of pain by loss of sensation.

Antibiotics: Drugs that kill microorganisms.

Antibody: A substance that is produced by the body from exposure to an antigen and triggers an immune response to fight infection.

Antigens: Substances, such as microorganisms or proteins found on the surface of blood cells, that can induce an immune response and cause the production of antibodies.

Apgar Score: A measurement of a baby's response to birth and life on its own, taken 1 and 5 minutes after birth.

Areola: The darker skin around the nipple.

Auscultation: A method of listening to the fetal heartbeat, either with a special stethoscope or the use of an ultrasound device.

Biophysical Profile: A means of measuring the fetus's breathing, muscle tone, body movement, and amount of amniotic fluid to check on the progress of pregnancy.

Braxton–Hicks Contractions: False labor pains.

Breech Presentation: The positioning of the fetus's buttocks or feet at the top of the birth canal.

Cephalopelvic Disproportion: A condition in which a baby is too large to pass through the mother's pelvis during delivery.

Chancre: An infectious sore caused by syphilis and appearing at the place of infection.

Chorioamnionitis: Inflammation of the membrane surrounding the fetus.

Chloasma: The darkening of areas of facial skin during pregnancy.

Chorionic Villi: Small sprouts that grow from the wall of the fertilized egg and develop into the placenta.

Colostrum: A fluid secreted from the breasts at the beginning of milk production.

Congenital Disorder: A condition that affects a fetus before it is born.

Contraction Stress Test: A test in which mild contractions of the mother's uterus are induced and the response of the fetus's heart rate is recorded.

Dilation and Curettage (D&C): A procedure in which the opening to the cervix is widened and tissue is gently scraped or suctioned from the lining of the uterus.

Doppler: A form of ultrasound that reflects motion—such as the fetal heartbeat—in the form of sounds.

Ectopic Pregnancy: A pregnancy in which the fertilized egg begins to grow in a place other than inside the uterus, usually in the fallopian tubes.

Edema: Swelling caused by fluid retention.

Electronic Fetal Monitoring: A procedure in which instruments are used to record the heartbeat of the fetus and contractions of the mother's uterus during labor.

Epidural Block: Anesthesia that numbs the lower half of the body.

Episiotomy: A surgical incision made in the perineum (the region between the vagina and the anus) to widen the vaginal opening for delivery.

Estrogen: A female hormone produced in the ovaries.

Fibroids: Growths that form on the inside of the uterus, on its outer surface, or within the uterine wall itself.

Follicle-Stimulating Hormone (FSH): A hormone produced by the pituitary gland that helps an egg to mature and be released.

Forceps: Special instruments placed around the baby's head to help guide it out of the birth canal during delivery.

Gamete Intrafallopian Transfer (GIFT): A treatment for infertility in which eggs are removed from a woman's ovary, mixed with the man's sperm, and placed into the fallopian tube to achieve pregnancy.

Glucose: A sugar that is present in the blood and is the body's main source of fuel.

Human Chorionic Gonadotropin (hCG): A hormone produced by the placenta once the fertilized egg has developed and attached to the uterine wall; its detection is the basis for most pregnancy tests.

Hydramnios: A condition in which there is an excess amount of amniotic fluid in the sac surrounding the fetus.

Insulin: A hormone that controls the levels of glucose (sugar) in the blood.

In Vitro Fertilization: A procedure in which an egg is removed from a woman's ovary, fertilized in a dish in a laboratory with the man's sperm, and then reintroduced into the woman's uterus to achieve a pregnancy.

Jaundice: A buildup of bilirubin that causes a yellowish appearance.

Laparoscopy: A surgical procedure in which a slender, light-transmitting instrument is used to view the pelvic organs.

Lecithin/Sphingomyelin (L/S) Ratio: Substances in the amniotic fluid that are measured to determine whether the fetus is mature enough to survive outside the uterus.

Linea Nigra: A line running from the navel to pubic hair that darkens during pregnancy.

Lochia: Vaginal discharge that occurs after delivery.

Luteinizing Hormone (LH): A hormone produced by the pituitary glands that helps an egg to mature and be released.

Macrosomia: A condition in which a fetus grows too large, often occurring when the mother is diabetic or in postterm pregnancy.

Meconium: A greenish substance that builds up in the bowels of a growing fetus and is normally discharged shortly after birth.

Miscarriage: Spontaneous loss of a pregnancy before 20 weeks.

Multiple Pregnancy: Carrying more than one fetus during pregnancy (twins).

Neural Tube Defect (NTD): A birth defect that results from improper development of the brain or spinal cord.

Nonstress Test: A test in which fetal movements felt by the mother or noted by the doctor are recorded, along with changes in the fetal heart rate.

Oxytocin: A drug used to help bring on contractions.

Paracervical Block: The injection of a local anesthetic into the tissues around the cervix to relieve pain during childbirth.

Perineum: The area between the vagina and the anus.

Pica: The urge to eat nonfood items during pregnancy.

Pituitary Gland: A gland located near the brain that produces hormones that cause an egg to mature and be released during ovulation.

Placenta: Tissue that connects mother and fetus and provides nourishment to and takes away waste from the fetus.

Placenta Previa: A condition in which the placenta lies very low in the uterus, partially or completely covering the opening.

Postterm Pregnancy: A pregnancy that extends beyond 42 weeks.

Preeclampsia: A condition of pregnancy in which high blood pressure, fluid retention, and protein in the urine are present.

Preterm: Born before 37 weeks.

Progesterone: A female hormone that is produced in the ovaries and prepares the lining of the uterus during the second half of the menstrual cycle to nourish a fertilized egg.

Pudendal Block: An injection given in the perineum that relieves pain during delivery but not labor.

Pyelonephritis: An infection of the kidney.

Quickening: The mother's first feeling of movement of the fetus.

Respiratory Distress Syndrome (RDS): A condition of some preterm babies in which the lungs are not fully developed.

Retracted Nipple: A nipple that has pulled inward.

Spina Bifida: A neural tube defect that results from improper closure of the fetal spinal column.

Spinal Block: A form of anesthesia that numbs the lower half of the body.

Stillbirth: Delivery of a fetus who has died before birth.

Sudden Infant Death Syndrome (SIDS): The sudden death of a baby for no apparent reason.

Tachycardia: Rapid heart beat.

Teratogens: Agents that can cause birth defects when a woman is exposed to them during pregnancy.

Transducer: A device that emits sound waves and translates the echoes into electrical signals used in ultrasound.

Trimester: Any of the three 3-month periods into which pregnancy is divided.

Tubal Ligation: A method of female sterilization in which the fallopian tubes are closed by tying, banding, clipping, or sealing with electric current.

Ultrasound: A test in which sound waves are used to produce images to examine the fetus or view the internal organs.

Umbilical Cord: A cord-like structure that connects the fetal blood vessels to the placenta.

Vacuum Extraction: The use of a special instrument attached by suction to the baby's head to help guide it out of the birth canal during delivery.

Vasectomy: A method of male sterilization in which a portion of the vas deferens is removed.

Vernix: The greasy, whitish coating of a newborn.

Index